S0-BPO-802

MARY
LOUISE

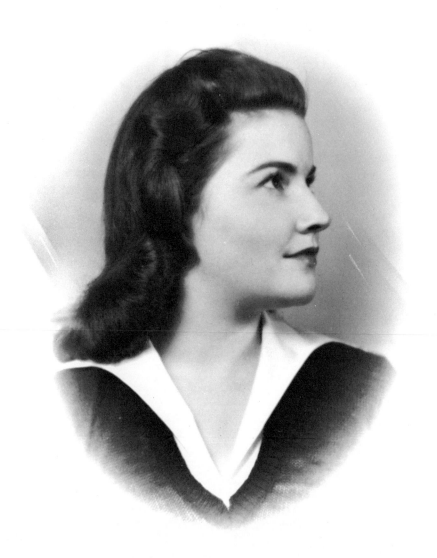

MARY LOUISE

LYLE STUART

The Citadel Press
Secaucus, New Jersey

First Edition
Copyright © 1972 by Lyle Stuart
All rights reserved
Published by Citadel Press, Inc.
A subsidiary of Lyle Stuart, Inc.
120 Enterprise Avenue, Secaucus, N.J. 07094
In Canada: George J. McLeod Limited
73 Bathurst St., Toronto 2B, Ontario
Manufactured in the United States of America
Library of Congress catalog card number: 76-186400
ISBN 0-8065-0282-7

NOTE

The newspaper is called *The Independent*. It appeared in September, 1969, with an unusual front page. The page was white except for a simple photograph of a soft, gentle-looking woman holding a lion cub in the zoo in Rome, 1964.

Somewhat below the photograph and to the right, was the statement:

> Mary Louise Stuart, co-founder with her husband, Lyle, of *The Independent*, died of cancer at 1 a.m. on Sunday, August 24, in Port Maria, Jamaica. She died in the arms of her husband. She was 46 years old.

Two years have passed and yet the demand for copies of the newspaper has not diminished.

What follows is a reprint of the entire issue of that newspaper with some additions and an afterword.

PROEM

Why publish this in book form?

Vanity? No. I am long past that.

Why then?

To inspire others? Perhaps. Perhaps this little book will give hope to someone somewhere so he or she can continue to believe that there can indeed be a genuinely happy marriage.

But that's an excuse.

To show that one-to-one man-woman relationships can work out for a lifetime? There is so little of true love in the world today, that this would be a demonstration made by a fool for fools.

Why then?

Perhaps because this radiant woman was too precious to die unknown and unsung.

So that as long as there is a copy of this book anywhere in the world and someone to read it, she will live a little longer—if only in memory. . . .

LYLE STUART

Port Maria,
Jamaica, W.I.

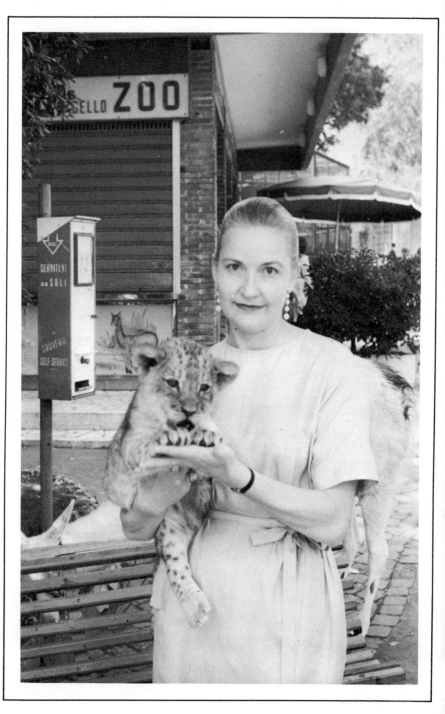

FOR OUR SON, RORY JOHN,
AND OUR DAUGHTER, SANDRA LEE

C HANCE—some call it fate—is sometimes
a mystical, beautiful thing. Your mother
and I often talked about the tenuous circumstances that brought us together.

It began this way. And it was crowded with
"ifs". . . .

If C. D. Russell, creator of the "Pete the Tramp"
comic strip, hadn't visited Halloran Hospital that
day during World War II to cheer up the soldiers
in the hospital wards, he and I would not have met.
We spent no more than ten minutes together, and
although we spoke to each other on the phone
some months later, we never met again.

During those ten minutes, he learned that I had
written and had published some articles about the
war. He suggested that, after my discharge, I join
the Hearst organization. If not for him, I might
not have applied to Hearst's International News
Service for a reporter's job.

Russell arranged an interview for me with Barry
Farris of I.N.S. Farris offered me a job in my

choice of three cities. If I "worked out," he promised to reassign me to New York.

I tended to favor Pittsburgh. If not for Harold O. Warren, Jr., who, until his recent retirement, edited *Family Circle*, I would not have selected Columbus, Ohio.

"Go to Columbus," he said over a lunch in Stouffer's restaurant on Fifth Avenue. "It is the most typical of American cities, and you'll get a genuine feel of the Midwest."

I had been in Columbus for just a few weeks. I was in my early twenties—very ambitious—and totally without resources except for those within myself. And I had already kicked up a storm with "scoops" about such things as a split in the American Legion, corruption in the local medical association, and various and sundry other stories that attracted more than I.N.S.'s usual share of space in the Ohio papers.

An interview I did with Mae West in her bedroom, when she appeared in person in *Catherine Was Great* in Columbus, was picked up on both the national and international I.N.S. wires. I received two raises in two months and was about to receive a third.

To earn some extra money, I also became the Columbus stringer for *Variety*, the show-business weekly. This, coupled with my being from New

York, gave me a "hot shot" glamour in provincial Columbus that I really didn't deserve.

I dropped in to see O. Joe Olson that day. He was managing editor of the Ohio State University *Alumni Monthly* and we had met when I went to the campus to do a story on the betatron—an atom smasher. (The story, which was widely published, brought the F.B.I. in full force to Columbus. For this was before the world knew we had the atom bomb—and information about atom-smashing was "top secret.")

Olson introduced me to his boss, Jack Fuller. We had some pleasant conversation and I made ready to leave. Olson said he was leaving too and would walk across the campus with me.

We walked across the campus toward High Street, where we would go our separate ways. Halfway, Olson met a professor and stopped to talk. I politely moved out of earshot. The conversation dragged on and I tried to catch Olson's eye to wave goodbye. He was too engrossed in talk. Three times I resolved to go and three times I hesitated.

If I had gone, I might never have known Mary Louise.

It was unlikely that I would see Olson again. We didn't have any personal relationship. He seemed like a warm, very witty fellow. But I was a high school dropout with not very much respect for formal education and he was an alumnus-loving, football-team-cheering, rah-rah university man.

That I waited was quite out of character for me. Perhaps it was my loneliness . . . the deep, melancholy loneliness that had always been my companion. . . .

"Man is forever lonely
there can be no time or circumstances in all
his days to lead him out of his loneliness.
His ways are those of clouds and tides.
Not even he who seeks the crowded solace
of the street
Can hope to find a single comrade there. . . ."

Olson rejoined me at last. He apologized for detaining me. Then, as we shook hands as if to part, he invited me to join him for a few beers at a campus hangout called Larry's. I am not much of a drinker but I said okay. Then he asked if it was all right if his wife, Ruth, joined us and I said sure.

Joe and Ruth were tall, lanky Swedes. She was gentle and patient. He was gentle and earthy. He had a newspaper background. A big hunk of his income went for alcohol.

We liked each other, the Olsons and I, and we began to spend time together. The three of us were strangers in a provincial town, surrounded by provincial people.

I don't recall at what point the suggestion was made. I had known the Olsons a short time when they suggested that I meet a friend of theirs. Actually, they asked if I'd be "willing"—for it was understood that this wasn't to be a "date" in the usual sense of the word.

The young lady was the widow of Jack Buckler, who had been Joe's best friend. Buckler had been an Air Force pilot. A few weeks before, his plane had been hit by flak. He and the crew bailed out. His was the only parachute that failed to open.

Mary Louise Buckler was in mourning. Although she'd been putting up a brave front in public, they knew that the news had devastated her. The couple had been very much in love—and married less than six months. (She was to write some months later in a letter that she was probably the only serviceman's wife who hadn't worried about her husband because she was so sure he was coming back to her.)

For weeks after receipt of the War Department telegram notifying her of his death, she continued to receive his letters telling her how much he loved her, talking about their future life together. And then her letters to him began to come back—one or two a day—and a badly smashed package containing the crumbled remains of cookies she had baked for him.

The Olsons thought I might cheer her up. I said I would try.

The four of us met at the Olson place and then went to dine at a restaurant called the Jai Lai. She was a strikingly attractive natural redhead. The word "beautiful" is much overused, but beautiful she was—with a radiance that shone through her quiet sorrow.

I was my then-self: bold, superficially confident, dogmatic. Instinct told me that the worst thing to do was to show sympathy for her plight. So I tried to anger her.

"You were a pretty smart-alecky kid who took the view that, if somebody was smart enough, they wouldn't get killed," she said on a tape we made last May. "So, of course, I argued this point with you a good deal."

"—And your red hair turned redder and you were infuriated. Right?" I remarked in the same taped conversation.

"No, I wasn't. Because I just thought you were a smart-alecky kid. I wasn't that emotionally moved by your viewpoint, of course."

She laughed and added: "You'll never know how surprised I was when I walked into the Olsons' and saw you for the first time. You happened to look more like a kid than most people of that age [22] looked, and I was just a little shocked to see they had produced someone so immature."

"And then what happened?" I asked. "And then, right after the Jai Lai, I escorted you home. Right?"

Mary Louise giggled. "Yes, you did. That was very gallant of you." She added, "It wasn't very far away. Where I roomed was about two blocks from where you roomed, and it was a very nice, mild spring evening."

"And then, on the doorstep, you turned and said 'It's been nice' and bid me goodbye, right?"

"Right."

"And that was that. And then, I think the next time I saw you—it was in the Olsons' attic—"

"—They were probably still matchmaking," Mary Louise interjected, "because they called to ask me over or I called to ask if it was all right to come over and you were either right there or they knew you were coming—but they didn't mention this to me."

"No, but I knew that you were coming so I kind of hung around. But then when you came in, you didn't even say hello to me—"

"Well, you and Joe were playing chess and I didn't want to interrupt you—"

"No, no. The room was about as big as a closet."

"Yes, that was a very small attic apartment that they had."

"And there we were, the four of us, and you didn't even say hello—so I got up and left."

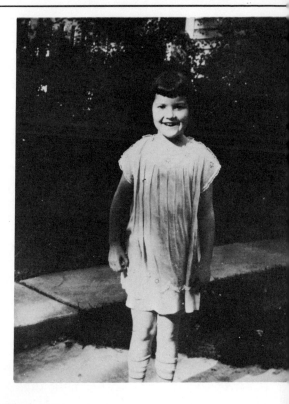

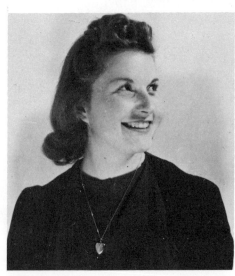

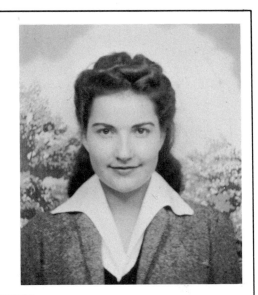

(Left) At Grandma's house in Toledo, which she visited every summer

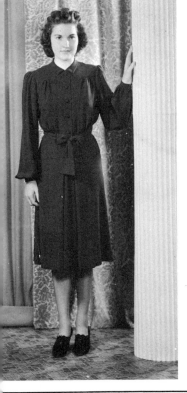

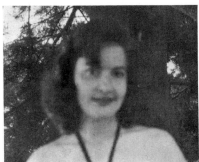

A couple of weeks later, Ruth Olson mentioned that Mary Louise had been dating a soldier from Georgia who was stationed on campus in a military training program of some sort.

As my "status" rose in Columbus, girls had become plentifully available. I was usually involved in two or three "romances" at any given time. And yet the echo of my meeting with Mary Louise stayed with me and bothered me.

I shared a room with a University student in an approved rooming house across from the campus. There was a public telephone in the hall and one day I found myself using it to phone Mary Louise. I talked with a southern accent, pretended that I was from Georgia, and expressed surprise that she didn't know me by my voice. She continued to insist that I identify myself.

Finally, reluctantly, I abandoned the act. I told her who I was. There was what seemed to me a long, long pause and I fully expected her to hang up.

"Why don't you buy me a Coke?" she said at last.

I think I began to fall in love with her at that moment. I have never stopped loving her since.

". . . *nor yet in secret bonds of love can man forget*
his heart's own solitude
Though lips may meet

and hand touch hand in intimate embrace
a stranger still abides within the mind
no word can reach . . . no vision ever trace.
A lonely god, enthroned in lonely space
fashioned us out of silence as we are
as single as a tree
as separate as a star."

Anderson Scruggs wrote the poem "Man Is Forever Lonely" and I quoted from it, with permission, in my first published book, a novel called
God Wears a Bow Tie.

I was a lonely, neurotic youth, reaching for goals
unknown, hungering for something I couldn't de-
fine, struggling to understand the world about me
and my place in it.

This was not the face I showed to the world, but
it was my face. We all wear an eternal mask, and
beneath mine were the doubts and indecisions of
a young man who had lived part of his teen years
on welfare and who felt keenly the atavistic fear of
being without job and thus without bread and the
bread of life itself, self-respect.

It was my boss at I.N.S. speaking: "That girl
you had at the Dugout. You know: that redhead.
What a build! What a face! Isn't she the doll who
won the Miss Columbus contest?"

My ego feasted on comments like that. I was
young enough and foolish enough to be proud that

other people found her so attractive. I admired her for all the wrong reasons.

We were worlds apart in our backgrounds. My father was an atheist who left Vienna in rebellion against his father's orthodox Jewishness. He committed suicide when I was six. Within another six years I had found my own way to atheism.

She had grown up on an Ohio farm, the daughter of Methodist parents who had alternated between farming and schoolteaching.

It was 1945. In Columbus, Ohio, black people were still commonly referred to as "niggers" and Jews were little more than "white niggers" and both were scorned as much but no more than the British.

From an early age—far ahead of my time, I think —I had come to realize that the key to a person may be found in his racial attitudes. I had two close friends back in New York City: Joe Whalen, who was Irish and an ex-Catholic, and Avant Keels, who was black. I felt strongly against racism in any form.

She and I sat on the porch hammock. We were in the dark with only the distant street lamps casting their dim glow.

I had decided to test her.

"There's something I think I'd better tell you," I said.

"What's that?"

I decided to go all the way. "I'm part Negro," I said.

Thirty seconds passed in stilled silence and then she reached for my hand. "That doesn't matter," she said quietly.

There were the girls from the sorority houses. There was Greta who worked for United Press and Charlotte who worked for I.N.S. There were waitresses and secretaries and the eligible daughters of state executives. But somehow my dates with them seemed dull. They all seemed to be cut from the same master recording. They were all quite predictable. They were all impressed with the young newspaper reporter who was creating so much excitement in Columbus. All, that is, except for Mary Louise.

One morning when she was free (she had now returned to classes at Ohio State University) I invited her to attend the Governor's press conference with me.

I thought I would impress her. I knew that Governor Frank Lausche liked me and would be especially gracious to any girl I thought enough of to escort to his conference. He was. He held both of her hands, looked into her eyes, and told her how lovely she was and how, as long as she was with me, she'd be welcome any time.

That day I decided to show off. I had been pressing the Governor for days about whether or not he intended to sign a bill. The bill would have increased the deposit on beer bottles and given the brewers some $14,000,000. The bill had been passed unanimously by the legislature.

The Governor had asked me to remain with him after the conference the day before. When we were alone he asked me what the bill was all about and why I was so interested in it. I explained that I thought it was a corrupt piece of legislation, aimed against the public purse, and bought vote by vote by the brewers.

Now, with Mary Louise sitting next to me, I asked him again—referring to the bill only by number.

"Governor Lausche, have you decided what you're going to do about bill eleven fourteen?"

The press conference was just about to end. He knew what he was doing to the other newsmen present, for there was a twinkle in his eye when he said, "Yes, Lyle, I have decided to veto it in the public interest."

The other reporters crowded around him. "What bill? What is the bill about, Governor?" Pandemonium had broken loose.

I took Mary Louise by the hand and went to the press phones. I dictated my story to the I.N.S. office. And all the while, the other reporters were frantically trying to learn what the bill was all about.

It was a neat scoop. The story made banner headlines in more than sixty Ohio papers. It was a "we interrupt this program to bring you a special bulletin" item on the local radio stations. Once again, I.N.S. had thoroughly trounced the A.P. and the U.P.

My story had made so clear the corrupt origins and intent of the legislation that, when the bill was sent back to the legislature, there was a unanimous vote to uphold the Governor's veto. Even the men who had sponsored the measure now no longer dared to vote for it.

I assumed that Mary Louise would be impressed.

Her parents drove in from the farm outside of Milford Center to visit her in Columbus that weekend. I saw her on the following morning.

"Did you tell your folks about meeting the Governor?" I asked.

"No," she said. "I didn't think of it."

"Well, didn't you mention it to your landlady or to your friend Rita?"

"No," she said, somewhat amused.

I was a little shaken. I had done what seemed to me an impressive thing. Any other girl on campus would have boasted to everyone that she'd met the Governor. Mary Louise hadn't bothered to mention it.

It appeared that our values were far, far apart.

Beneath her youthful beauty were qualities so remarkable that I struggled to understand some of
them and couldn't fathom others. She was all
woman: luscious, tempting, pliable, and respon-
sive. But she had such a fresh, wholesome manner
that the paradox of her quiet courage and her iron
will, her brilliant and perceptive mind, her sense
of justice, and her ability to see things so clearly
and in perfect context were too much for me to
believe. To further confound me, she was totally
without pretensions.

When I made a pass at her in a downtown movie
theatre, she looked about shyly and said, "Not
here." Later, when I was covering the I.N.S. office
on a Saturday night, she asked, "Can you leave
here for a while and not get into trouble?"

"Sure," I said.

"Then why don't you take me to a hotel room
and make love to me?"

One afternoon I got a clue. We were on the bus
going downtown, each on separate missions. I had
the morbid and unpleasant task of witnessing and
reporting on the electrocution of two Negroes who
had recently been convicted of murdering a 73-
year-old jeweler in Cincinnati.

Somehow, the conversation turned to her folks.
In response to something I said, she assured me

that her father had not been away from her mother for a single night since they were married.

A little bell sounded in my brain. I had no intentions of marrying. But I knew that, if I ever did, it would be to someone who came from a family where the parents were devoted to each other. I believed (and believe) that we tend to imitate our parents . . . tend to play out the same dramas in our own lives.

One day we were to meet in front of Long's Book Shop at 15th and High Streets.

I was there first. And then I saw her, and she came toward me, her arms pressing her schoolbooks against her breast, and she was smiling her warm, radiant smile at me.

Twenty-four years have passed—nearly a quarter of a century—and there are thousands of indelible impressions of her locked in my memory. But always, when I close my eyes and think "Mary Louise," the first picture that comes to mind is the memory of her walking toward me that day— my beautiful redhead with her beautiful smile.

I was a young man on the move. When I.N.S. failed to keep its promise to recall me to New York for "bigtime" reporting, I resigned.

I returned to New York. There was a phone message asking me to come immediately to the I.N.S. office. There was also a special-delivery letter asking me to see Abel Green of *Variety*.

In a letter dated July 26, 1945, Mary Louise wrote in part:

"Last night, as I was leaving the house for dinner, my landlady asked if there were a message in case someone should call me. I replied sadly, 'No, no message—he won't call.' She said, 'Oh, you're going to be lonesome for a while.' I could but sigh yes.

"My sociology instructor excused us from class today and tomorrow. He's spending an extended weekend in Kansas City. I was tempted to tell him (but I refrained from telling him) that he picked a helluva time to go. He must have known that you are gone and I no longer mind arising for a nine o'clock. . . . Also, it seems like more than a coincidence that my landlady should be going out of town this weekend. . . . You timed your departure very badly, My Love.

"Everything is as it was before you left—except that you are gone. And that makes everything different. The heat is more oppressive. Classes are less interesting. I am tired now. . . ."

I was to see her again sooner than I'd expected. I joined *Variety* in August at twice the salary I'd been making with Hearst, and I managed to maneuver so that my first important assignment was

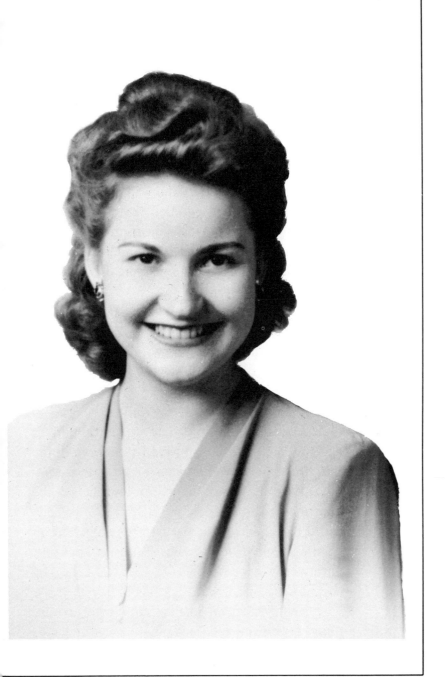

to return to Columbus, Ohio, for the world premiere of *Captain Eddie,* a 20th Century-Fox film
based on the life of Eddie Rickenbacker.

Just before I knew I was returning to Columbus,
she had written: "This day . . . without you . . . is
almost over. I will be glad when days are different
—when I cling to moments and want them to last."

In response to my suggestion that she just pack
up and leave everything and join me in New York:
"My present state of mind is not such that I can
give you the promised enumeration of considera-
tions and complications.

"To do that, I will have to be alone without
interruption for awhile. I want it to be soon. I need
to think. I think about it now, all the time, but
each thought conflicts with the thought before
and I am in a daze. Suffice it to say that I love
you dearly. Of that I am sure."

The *Captain Eddie* premiere was an important
event in Columbus. There were banners on all the
main streets. The front pages of all three newspapers were devoted almost exclusively to the
"celebrities" who were flying in from everywhere.
Even the leading restaurants were serving water in
special *Captain Eddie* glasses, furnished by 20th
Century-Fox.

My *Variety* review was supposed to be one of the
key reviews, but I paid small attention to the film.
I found myself, instead, looking at her.

Another parting. And there were her letters to look forward to.

August 3, 1945

"Dear Lyle,

"It was much better to have your letter to come home to than have nothing at all. I forgave you its brevity—but only because you had told me meanwhile what you've been doing. Hereafter, except in the instance that you expect to appear in Columbus, enlighten me as to your activities. I want to know what you do. To read about what you do is an inadequate substitute for doing what you do. But I prefer even the substitute with its inadequacy to nothing at all.

"Aside from, and over and above, and completely beyond that was your implication that you love me much. And that was my solace, last night."

Two pages later, the letter ended with:

"It seems to me as if I have practically outdone myself in writing at such length. And I've said very little of real import. But there's little of real import that I can say except that I love you. I love you."

August 7, 1945

"Today has been eventful and joyous," she wrote, "all because I received your letter of Saturday the loneliest in the week night. Until I received that letter, I had been brooding upon ways and means to teach you a lesson about not writing to me. . . ."

August 10, 1945

"Having received your second Variety gripe—that of 8 Aug 45—I begin to wonder if you like working for Variety. And then again, I wonder if you would ever like working for anyone. And I doubt it. Shall we retire to an atoll?"

August 13, 1945

". . . I know not if my apathy is to be attributed to the weather; or to my realization of a job not well done insofar as intellectual pursuits are concerned; or to exhaustion resulting from mental conflict; or to your farness. (Underneath it all, I know it's your farness. It is with considerable reluctance that I confess that. I thereby place myself at a disadvantage. Imagine that! No bargaining power!) "

August 13, 1945

"Dear Lyle,

"I am dismayed by my irrepressible urge to write to you oftener than you deserve. It's very unlike me. Usually I write to people less often than they deserve. Perhaps that's because most people are more deserving than you.

"There I go being catty again. Actually, all this is because I want to see you and to talk to you and to. Writing to you is a heluva substitute. I must swear off. It's getting like a drinking habit. . . ."

August 14, 1945

"You can always remember this as the day Japan surrendered and I wrote to you three times.

"I have been unable to enter fully into the spirit of the occasion. My late husband is not coming back and my next husband is in New York which is very far away when measured in inches, one of which would be too far away. . . . Gee, what am I now? Love making?

". . . there are some things we should discuss before I come to New York. . . . First and foremost, do you think I should plan to stay? I mean rationally, weighing pros and cons, do you? . . . .

"Besides the pleasure, delight and sheer joy of being together sometimes, we will get to know each other better. That I regard as essential before embarking upon marriage, whether you do or not. Maybe you think not because you think you know me well enough already—which maybe you do and maybe you don't. But I don't think I know you well enough. . . ."

August 21, 1945

"Dear Lyle,

"I am disheveled and disabled and convinced that tennis should be played frequently or not at all. . . . Oh well, I'll probably be able to move without pain again in a few days.

". . . I'm well aware of the deficiencies of poor Columbus. And somewhat aware of the attributes of New York (although I haven't gone so far as to embrace the crowds on Broadway). But, My Love, there are beauties even in Columbus on nights like tonight. It's the sort of night when people should be loving. . . ."

Three letters later, on August 25, 1945:

"I would prefer to be in New York with you tonight—or to have you in Columbus with me—or to be almost anywhere together. . . .

". . . the only other query that you've made that remains unanswered (except for your offhand, indirect and too too subtle inquiries about when I'm coming to New York) is the one about your project of 1 Aug 45. Take a deep breath. This will come as a considerable disappointment to you. No Jr."

And the postscript:

"Why don't you sometime tell me that you desperately want and need me. Or do you?"

Our courtship was erratic. She came to New York to live with a friend. For a while, we lived together in Brooklyn Heights on Montague Street in the apartment of a former high school teacher of mine who was going on vacation and who thought we were married. From our window we could see the old penny bridge—since torn down.

I left *Variety* to become editor of a looks-like-*Time* music magazine. It was concerned with the

Big Bands and songs and songwriters and music publishers and singers and a new creature on the scene known as "the disk jockey."

Gene Fowler wrote for *Music Business,* as did Fred Allen and Philip Wylie.

My editorials suggested to the publishing industry that the future of sheet music lay in a program that would put a "$100 piano" into every home in America.

I wrote editorials warning that these Johnny-come-lately "disk jockies" would soon become the most important element in "making a song hit" and that the importance of the band and the singer would soon fade. (We formed an organization called The American Society of Disk Jockeys.)

I offended distant members of my family who had an interest in RCA by attacking "General" David Sarnoff and his attempt to inflict 45-rpm records as the new way, when it was obvious to me that Columbia's 33⅓-rpm was more practical and would, in time, triumph. It did.

When the time came to give up the Montague Street apartment, I returned to my mother's little apartment in Flatbush, and Mary Louise moved in with a friend in Queens.

We had dates almost every evening. But, as I became more engrossed in my work, I tended to take her for granted. She'd come to my office in the old CBS building and often I would keep her waiting for hours while I caught up on the work that I should have done at the typewriter during the day. She never complained. She would play the piano in the outer room. Or she would sit quietly and patiently watching me.

She charmed everyone without trying. Once, when we were backstage at a function at Carnegie Hall, songwriter Frank Loesser couldn't keep his eyes off her. (He was to go on to write *Guys and Dolls* and *The Most Happy Feller.*)

He asked me if she was "taken." I laughed and said there was no harm in trying.

He chatted with her at length, but then, when he tried to arrange a date, she pointed across to me.

"You know Lyle, don't you?" she asked.

"Sure," he said. "We're friends."

"Well, I belong to him."

Flattering to me, but I had come to take it all for granted and my casual treatment of her took its toll. Five months later, she left New York. She visited her folks (who had retired to Florida) and then her sister, Eileen, in Akron.

She settled in Akron. She became involved in an embryonic political movement. To support herself, she got a job with the telephone company. The men flocked about like flies and two proposed to her.

I flew to Ohio. We stayed together for a few days while I earnestly tried to persuade her to return to New York. Now, at last, I was willing to make the "grand sacrifice"—I would marry her.

She said no.

Nothing I could say would move her. I spent half my weekly salary on long-distance phone calls.

March, 1946. April. May.

On May 4, she wrote: ". . . I've nothing of considerable significance to relate. I'm the same woman. Except a few days older. You know, grass and dandelions flourishing on the nourishment of my decomposing body—a few days nearer that.

"Worse, I haven't been living. Preparing to live though. That's pretty important. People can't live all the time.

"Guess no one quite comprehends my preparation, the indirection of it all. Maybe you do, partly. But you think it's absurd. So be it. . . .

"I have no idea that you're interested in the foregoing choice bits of information. Nor do you want to hear my account of my social activities. Nor can I talk about you, not knowing what you've been doing or anything. It occurs to me that this is an unfair arrangement. Request that we alternate on dates for writing. E.g., next month you write between the first and fifth."

Although the letter was signed "With love," I

didn't rush to respond. I had not concealed my dislike of the political crowd she was with, or they for me. They were opposed to "success" in our society—and to anyone who sought it on any level.

Days passed. Interviews with songwriter Leo Robin: ("Jerry Kern? He was a terribly nasty person. I would hand him a lyric and if he didn't like it, he'd toss it onto the floor. . . .")

Sitting in a penthouse with Johnny Mercer and Harold Arlen while they composed the score for their forthcoming hit show, *St. Louis Woman.*

Stopping Ethel Merman's rehearsal for *Annie Get Your Gun* while my staff photographer took pictures of Richard Rodgers, Oscar Hammerstein, and Irving Berlin standing together in the empty orchestra. (With Berlin griping, "Stopping the show like this is costing us money!" Berlin, the opium smoker, who, when he rose from being a singing waiter at Coney Island to a multimillionaire songwriter, once learned that a fellow former-waiter was down on his luck and waiting in the outer room hoping for a five-dollar handout. Berlin slipped out the back way, where, to his embarrassment, he ran face on into the fellow he was trying to duck. "Irving," the friend said, "I want you to know, you're one fellow about whom they can truly say, 'Success hasn't changed him a bit.' ")

Lunching with Mayor O'Dwyer, ex-Mayor Jimmy Walker, and film star Pat O'Brien at Toots Shor's.

Listening to Harold Rome explain why he wrote *Call Me Mister*. ("After the dread and horror of the war years, I thought people were ready for a happy show.")

Two weeks passed. I was trying to fill my life, but even though I was sometimes going "around the clock," it seemed empty and my "success" purposeless.

And then, on May 18, she wrote,

". . . Grieved to note your delinquency in your scheduled correspondence with me. Needless to say, I'd like a letter from you."

The letter was signed, "Exceedingly sincerely, Mary Louise."

My mood soared that day. I had tried to forget her by immersing myself in work and by dating all the pretty girls with the pretty faces and the pretty bodies and the blank minds. And it hadn't worked.

I knew that I was competing with her Akron suitors. They were aggressive. And they were there.

It took weeks before I could persuade her by letter and phone to schedule a weekend in New York with me. A few days before she was to arrive, she wrote in part:

"It's very hot and I yearn to be swimming or playing tennis.

"Since I scheduled next weekend with you, I've been engaged in frenzied futile efforts to find some garments to wear. Everything I came upon that was worth having was quite out of my budget. Consequently, in desperation I bought material and a pattern after work yesterday and set upon the project of making a suit. I sewed until four this morning. . . ."

She had once won a national 4-H contest and a memorable trip to Chicago when, as a girl on the farm, she sewed her own complete outfit.

The telegram read: EXPECT TO ARRIVE AT 3:44 FRIDAY AFTERNOON. BETTER BE THERE BOY. ALSO BETTER TRY TO MAKE A RETURN RESERVATION SUNDAY HERE OR TO CLEVELAND. AKRON TRAVEL AGENCY IS SOMEWHAT DILITANT.

We rented a large bright room on a high floor in the Lincoln Hotel and had a delightful weekend, except for those moments when conversation strayed to the differences in our attitudes about the American big-business system.

And then, all too quickly it was over and she was on a train back to Akron.

On Monday, there was another telegram: THOUGHT YOU MIGHT LIKE TO KNOW THAT I ARRIVED HOME INTACT. AND THAT I FIND AKRON AND OHIO BELL AT LEAST SLIGHTLY SORDID TODAY. LOVE. MARY LOUISE.

A series of letters from me, trying to convince her that she was making a mistake in Ohio. Trying to persuade her to live with me and be my love.

But the differences in our attitudes on many things had crystallized. On July 20, she could write:

". . . I realize that you too are not entirely responsible for your actions at this time. There has arisen a condition conducive to irrationality. I can't wholeheartedly condemn you for contradictory manifestations.

"I know that you want me—that my failure to respond is painful to you. Aside from—here's my confession—aside from the urgency of my remaining here until our initial step in the election campaign has been completed, I remain away because I want to hurt you.

"I want you too, but not with the unreserved kind of want that should compose love. I'll never want you that way, I'll never wholly love you, our marriage will never be more than a 'possibly temporary thing' until you become conscious—until you see things as they are and not as a fantasy resultant of the myth. . . . You assure me you have no political convictions. But every sentiment you've ever voiced has indicated your belief in the desirability of living the kind of life prescribed in the myth.

"Apparently, you base your belief on this premise—that individual righteousness and progress such as can be made according to the capacity of each is the solution.

"You believe that each person controls his own destiny. The latter, if you recall, was your main topic of conversation the first night we met. You have never retracted any part of that conversation. . . . You fluff off reality. Circumstances have forced me to face reality. I should think that your father's final disillusionment would have effected some sort of honest thought on your part. But no, you go on in your dream world aiding and abetting conditions that will, in all probability, bring even you with your extraordinary perceptions and talent, to disaster. . . ."

Our head-on conflict because of my rigid conservatism seemed insurmountable.

But something drew us together despite the doubts and the indecisions, and late in July, still expressing strong intellectual reservations, she agreed to marry me.

I couldn't quite believe it. Her sister was strongly opposed to me. Her political companions considered me an enemy of what they stood for. Her two suitors in Akron had become more intense in trying to persuade her to choose one of them.

On July 30, she wired: PACKING TEMPO HIT NEW HIGH. PATH CLEARED THRU DINING ROOM. I'LL ARRIVE PER SCHEDULE. LOVE YOU LOVE YOU LOVE YOU LOVE YOU LOVE YOU LOVE. MARY LOUISE

On August 2, she wired: JUST CAME FROM MIL-
FORD CENTER WHERE I RECEIVED MANY BEST
WISHES, HOPE TO BE NEW YORK BOUND BY TOMOR-
ROW NIGHT. WILL WIRE TIME TOMORROW. LOVE.
MARY LOUISE

It seemed now that nothing could go wrong, for
I had come to know that I wanted and needed her
at my side more than I had ever wanted anything
in the world. And yet I knew of her own justified
doubts . . . and of the forces at work in Akron.

And then it came. On the evening of August
3, a wire which read: YOUR FEARS WERE WELL
FOUNDED. I CAN'T COME. THIS DECISION CRYSTALIZED
WITHOUT OUTSIDE INFLUENCE. I'VE CROSSED EVERY
BARRIER EXCEPT MY OWN FAILURE TO LOVE YOU.
PREVIOUS WORDS TO THE CONTRARY HAVE BEEN BUT
ATTEMPTS TO HELP BUILD THE HAPPY MARRIAGE
THAT YOU DESCRIBE. IT'S IMPOSSIBLE WITHOUT MY
LOVE. MY ONLY CONSOLATION FOR THE TRAGEDY OF
THIS IS MY REALIZATION THAT FUTURE SEPARATION
WOULD BE FAR MORE TRAGIC. BE ASSURED THAT MY
INDECISION IS OVER. IF HOWEVER YOU WANT FUR-
THER EXPLANATION WIRE ME AND I'LL CALL OR
WRITE AS YOU LIKE. MARY LOUISE

I walked the dark fringes of Prospect Park in
Brooklyn for three hours.

Later, I learned that her sister and one of her
Akron suitors had taken her to the train station,

convincing her all the while that she was making a most dreadful mistake. She had become ill, wired me, and then returned to her apartment, where she threw up in the bathroom.

I didn't sleep that night. I couldn't reconcile myself to losing her but there was nothing I could do but wait.

I hadn't long to wait. At 7:25 a.m. she wired me: ASHAMED AND AFRAID TO CALL YOU BUT I'M MISERABLE AND WILL COME IF YOU CAN FORGIVE ME. WIRE ME IF WHEN AND WHERE TO CALL. MARY LOUISE

We went to a wholesale jewelry house, where she selected her gold wedding band. It cost $14.

We were married in the Municipal Building in New York City.

She arrived minutes before the scheduled ceremony. She had been up all night sewing her wedding suit and hat.

My mother and my brother and my aunt were there for me. She was accompanied by a distant cousin by her first marriage.

The ceremony cost $3. It took five minutes. The date was September 26, 1946.

And so it began. With no apartment and no money. And I was between jobs. I had only her confidence in me to sustain me.

For the next year, my income was $100 a month

from the G.I. bill's "52-20" club. I stayed in our one-room flat with her—sharing a public bathroom. Forty of the $100 went to support my mother.

Mary Louise had two $1,500 war bonds. We lived on those. She also received a monthly check for about $28 as insurance compensation to her from the Veterans Administration for the loss of her first husband.

She didn't complain.

She was an excellent cook. She kept house. She turned our drab one room into a delightfully cozy place. We were together all the time.

In the April, 1940, issue of *Successful Farming*, there was a long article about her titled "Growing Up Gracefully" by Alfred W. Cherry.

In one paragraph, the writer described her as "an attractive auburn-haired lass who has just turned 17. She's a real farm girl, too, prepares all the meals for the family, makes nearly all her own clothes, and even helps her father in rush seasons by driving the tractor. But in spite of her very busy life she somehow always manages to achieve that look of just having stepped out of a bandbox."

She hadn't changed.

She made delightful meals when we entertained, and always on a budget of nickels and dimes.

Rather than have me seek a job, she encouraged me to try my hand at fiction. I sat at the typewriter in our one-room apartment, staring at the white sheet of paper.

"I can't get started," I said, after a blank hour.

"Write anything," she said. "You've got a writer's block."

I typed: "Here I am, staring at a white sheet of paper with nothing on it and—" when suddenly I was into the first sentence of what would become my only published novel.

We found a publisher. But he wouldn't meet my demands in terms of advance. We went to his office together to retrieve the script from his receptionist.

We walked along 57th Street, the script under my arm.

"I think it's time for me to go to work again," I said.

"Not if you don't want to," she said. "You're a very talented writer. If you want to write another novel, I'll go to work."

"No. I want you with me all the time. That's one of the things that was fun about being a novelist."

Nearly two years later, at an editorial conference, one of the publishing executives asked: "What ever became of that Lyle Stuart novel? It was never published."

Somehow they found me. I took the script from my drawer and they published *God Wears a Bow*

Tie. It went into three printings and then sold 240,000 in a paperback edition.

The book bore the simple dedication:

To Mary Louise

In the meantime, we were struggling to stay afloat.

A solution suggested itself. A former commanding officer of mine in the Air Transport Command also wanted to be a writer. He lived in Lynchburg, Virginia.

We agreed to move into his house and share living expenses. His wife and Mary Louise would take turns doing the household chores.

The couple came to New York at our invitation. Mary Louise and I both felt very strongly about the things human beings do to other human beings because of the difference in the shade of their skin.

My former C.O. and his wife met some of our black friends in social situations. They seemed to understand and agree with our point of view.

But no sooner had we moved our possessions into the house in Lynchburg, than there was a conference in the living room in which it was explained to us that what happens in New York was one thing but "this is the South and we have to live here."

It was the beginning of alienation.

In no time I had found my way into the black community. I was the second so-called "white man" to address the students at Dunbar High School.

Even the local C.I.O. made the mistake of inviting me to speak. The union was trying to organize the Craddock-Terry shoe workers. It was assumed that, as a newspaperman and writer, I'd talk union. Instead, I startled my audience by delivering a sermon on how they were defeating their own purpose by excluding Negroes from their organizing effort.

Mary Louise and I both wrote letters to the local newspaper. Pointing out that "both biology and the Bible agree that man is of one blood . . . etc."

In the context of today, it doesn't seem much. In the late 1940s, it was quite dramatic.

Madison Jones, Jr., who was then administrative secretary to Walter White (who headed the National Association for the Advancement of Colored People), was in constant correspondence with me. He expressed amazement that we were able to survive, concluding that perhaps it was Lynchburg's Quaker antecedents that kept me from being lynched for my open assault on the town's mores.

Mary Louise was with me every step of the way.

We were angered by a culture where a black man or woman could not try on a pair of gloves in the local shops—but would have to buy them and hope they fit. . . . Where no black person could enter the town's public library . . . where everything was separate and unequal.

We made many friends among the leaders of the black community. They cited as the worst humiliation the fact that there was no single standard. In one city, a black person could sit at one section of a Walgreen store's lunch counter. In the next town, he might be able only to buy something to take out. And in the town after that, he was not allowed to enter the store for any reason.

The local paper was owned by the family of then-Senator Carter Glass. It finally announced, editorially, that no further letters from either Mr. Lyle Stuart or Mrs. Lyle Stuart would be permitted in its columns.

That night a rock smashed through our bedroom window.

Mary Louise received obscene postcards.

She sat worrying about me when I was late. I would stand in front of the local candy store and argue with a group of young whites who couldn't believe that a white man would say the things I said, and couldn't understand my "cool" in discussing racial things with them in a relaxed fashion.

(Jackie Robinson had broken the color bar in baseball. The World Series was on, and he was playing for the Brooklyn Dodgers against the New

York Yankees. My ex-C.O.'s father said in his booming southern accent, "Ah never thought I'd be cheering for Yankees, but I'm sure cheering for Yankees now!")

The situation was edging toward violence. We decided it was time to leave. We bid goodbye to our black friends: the Reverend Morris Tynes, the William T. Jackson family, Mr. and Mrs. Seay, and the others. Then, quietly, at 2 a.m., we got to the train depot and took a local to New York.

We got lucky. We located and were able to sublet a tiny apartment in New York's Hell's Kitchen. It was three floors above a fruit stand at the corner of 39th Street and Ninth Avenue. The sublease was for nearly two years.

It was a slum neighborhood and a rough one but, except for a few isolated incidents, there was nothing to make us feel that it was dangerous to walk the streets.

Being on the top floor with no air conditioning and a tar roof above us, we often felt that we were living in an oven. On summer evenings when the rest of New York was cooling off, our apartment was suffering its nightly roast, as the heat came down from the roof.

To escape in the daytime, we became members of the Museum of Modern Art. We went there frequently and saw all their old movies. We got to know the painting collection pretty well.

Often we would also go to the penthouse where, for 75¢ each as members, we would fill up on afternoon tea and petite sandwiches.

Days that we didn't go there, we would sometimes go to air-conditioned movies.

We enjoyed being together tremendously. We used to ride the Staten Island ferry quite often on hot days. We would take the open-top double-decker Fifth Avenue buses up to Fort Tryon Park.

And, in our womblike apartment we had lots of company and did lots of entertaining.

There was a problem in our Ninth Avenue apartment, which we weren't aware of.

In retrospect, Mary Louise was sure it was a problem that caused some of her difficulties which she'd then been persuaded to believe were psychological.

"I recall during that period feeling dizzy when I went out into the street," she said on a tape we made in May of 1969. "And of course it was quite a challenge to walk across anywhere that I could walk across. I frequently met you at Times Square and I had a choice of walking through the garment district, where it was like running a gauntlet with these characters sitting there whistling and making remarks, or going on 42nd Street, which was terrible in a different way with all the perverts and everything. Always someone would start following me, muttering things under his breath, and I wasn't really equipped to handle it.

"I still don't think any of this was the cause of my dizziness. The little philodendron that I tried to grow, my first efforts to grow house plants—which made me think at the time that I wasn't good at house plants—were the key to the problem. They just died. Plants die if they're in a bad environment.

"When we left there and Helen Hymes took over her apartment again, she had a tendency to keep her windows closed more tightly than we did.

"Two days after she was back, she woke up in the middle of the night, realizing that there was something frightfully wrong. She staggered out the door and screamed for help and collapsed. It was carbon monoxide poisoning from the gas refrigerator. I think this had been causing me trouble for the nearly two years we lived there. I remember when we first moved there—the first day or two—both of us suffered from headaches. And, of course, we never ever dreamed that anything was wrong with the refrigerator."

Mary Louise added: "All of these experiences were all part of it, and we still had a lot of fun.

"I was about run ragged, I must say, because

that place was the dirtiest, filthiest place there ever ever was, and I was busy cleaning and vacuuming all the time—because everything was covered with soot. I was trying to keep up with you and go all the places you wanted to go and make my clothes and keep the filthy place clean and cook good meals for pennies—which is about all we had to spend. That was a terrible challenge too, because for me going down to the vegetable stands downstairs was very difficult on account of the over-friendly salesmen in these places. You always used to kid me about George's fruit stand. I had quite an adjustment to make to this city, I must say!"

At Christmas time and before the following Father's Day, Mary Louise worked at a temporary job at Brooks Brothers, selling gift certificates. She was the only female employee on the main floor —and a delightful sight she was.

Money remained in short supply, and we never knew for certain how we'd meet next month's rent.

I registered at the New School for Social Research under the G.I. Bill of Rights. (In one of my writing seminars, my nine classmates included seven who were to go on to success as published novelists, including William Styron [*The Revolt of Nat Turner*] and Mario Puzo [*The Godfather*].)

I became involved in New School's problems and somehow found myself student chairman of the fund-raising committee. Marshall Field II was my co-chairman, and Mary Louise and I visited his home.

He was one of the wealthiest men in America, but his carpet was torn and the furniture in his home was well used.

He was impressed with her. She was a smart-looking woman, and attracted attention wherever she went.

She was never ostentatious. She had exquisite taste but it was not related to price tags. For many years of our marriage, she designed and made all of her clothes.

In later years, when we became quite wealthy, she loved to travel with me and we stayed in luxury hotels. She enjoyed her custom-made slack suits that we would buy in Rome at Brioni's. She bought a variety of inexpensive coats.

In later years when we lived in a $124-a-month, 5½-room cooperative apartment, we allowed ourselves the luxury of owning two cars, both of them inexpensive little foreign models.

Friends couldn't understand how we could continue to live in our high-crime-rate slum area. Her only complaint about our apartment was that we simply didn't have enough storage space.

Powerfully built men were afraid to walk the streets of our neighborhood but she went out unafraid. Her fears and worries were not about herself, but rather about me and the children. She was always admonishing me to "drive carefully."

She didn't wear perfume. She wore very little make-up. Her attractiveness was natural. For the first twenty years of our marriage she didn't set foot inside a beauty parlor. Only during the past three years did she have her hair washed and cut and styled. The red had faded and become laced with gray but she wouldn't dye it and I wouldn't have wanted her to.

Perfumed scents bothered her. She may have been allergic to them. Our soap was unscented. Even the talcum powder she used was without scent.

When I first knew her, she was smoking two to three packs of cigarettes a day. But she had enough consideration for her father so that, when she visited him, she never smoked where he might become aware of it. Her father disapproved of smoking.

I did too. Heretofore, any girl who smoked cigarettes would automatically turn me off. But she smoked, and whatever she did seemed different and okay. Only after she took the pulse test and saw, conclusively, that she was allergic to cigarettes, did she determine to quit. But she would quit, she said, only on becoming pregnant.

When she became pregnant, she stopped cold. She never smoked another cigarette. And she developed a strong antipathy toward the odor of cigarette smoke.

From the day she stopped smoking, I have not permitted anyone to smoke in our home or in our office. There have been no exceptions.

She visited her folks in Florida.

"Dear Husband," she wrote.

"My letters to you aren't nice and literate like yours are to me. Guess that's cause I love you so much. I'll be glad when I'm home and can talk to you and kiss you. . . ."

And two pages later: "Don't know why I'm writing all this stuff, though, 'cause I'll call you tomorrow night. I just wrote this to tell you I love you and so you'd receive something in the mail from me.

"Hope you're being a good boy.

With much love,
Your Best Wife

"P.S. I miss you, Luvra Boy.

"P.S. xxxxxxx, etc."

Mary Louise went to work as a secretary. I obtained a job as editor of a weekly newspaper in the women's ready-to-wear field. I had a staff of sixteen reporters and artists—all female. It was mostly a matter of selecting.

An unhappy period in our relationship had begun.

A year later, in an agonizing appraisal of what had happened, she was to write:

"In our marriage we have had some problems and much happiness too. We were not bound by the dogma of conventional morals; we were bound only by love.

"There was a kind of understanding between us about our freedom to have whatever kind of relationship we wanted with other men and women. We both had enough faith in ourselves and each other to believe there could be no serious threat to our marriage. I had no desire for extra-marital affairs. Lyle seemed to me to be amoral enough in many respects to be uninhibited about having extra-marital sex, and I did not relish the thought. But this kind of understanding seemed to be absolutely essential for our happiness since Lyle does not respond well to restrictions of any kind. . . .

"Thus it was that when Lyle spent many hours out, over and above legitimate appointments, some of these many hours were spent with other women, and it was of no crucial concern to me. . . . I did ask emphatically many times that when he overstayed the time I expected him home by more than an hour, he call me. This was because I

WORRIED, not about who he was spending his time with or how, but about his safety. . . ."

She described my occasional late hours. "His work at the paper took so much of his time that we hardly saw each other. This seemed to be justifiable 'separation' which was eased by my feeling that the very long overtime hours were temporary.

"However, now his social hours out became significant for an additional reason. They were practically the only time that he and I could have had together. . . .

"The explanation was obvious—it holds true in most instances of extra-marital escapades, whatever form they may take: the ego is nourished. . . . In Lyle's case, I felt there was further justification. Intimate knowledge of people and participation in experiences of all kinds provide food for a writer of fiction.

"After this had been going on for awhile, it happened—it just *happened*, I did not bring it about deliberately, that another man began to grow fond of me. Had I been more conscious and completely principled I would not have allowed it to happen.

"However, apparently my ego needed nourishment, too. Or to quote from psychiatry, I was 'acting out hostility' toward Lyle. At any rate, I allowed the relationship to develop to precisely the stage where I felt he could be mine if I wanted him.

"Not for an affair—because that means nothing to a woman. Any unattached man is likely to be ready for a brief affair at least with any woman unless she is downright repulsive to him—and sometimes even then.

"This 'adventure' of mine had come about without my taking anything from Lyle. . . . I had not been unfaithful in terms of extra-marital sex. . . ."

I became aware of the "other man" one evening when my own date couldn't make it and I came home early. She arrived at 8:30. When I asked, she told me who she'd been with and where she'd been.

At first I was upset, but there was no crisis. Then I gave her my consent to go out any time she wanted.

It happened again, a few days later. I third-degreed her until she admitted that the fellow was falling in love with her. He was baffled and could not understand her interest in him, since she had told him she was happily married.

Put to the test, I found I could not stand the thought of sharing her.

She was willing to defer to my wishes—but only if we both agreed on a single standard. Either neither of us were to have extracurricular affairs or we were both free to have them. She would not tolerate the common American "double standard."

In her year-later recap, she wrote: "One of the promises I had made (and I never in my life have made a promise that I failed to keep) was that I would quit my job any day, at any time of the day, if he asked me to. This, despite the fact that it's a very traumatic thing for me to do anything unfair. Even on jobs where I have been very obviously exploited, I have given some notice. . . . On this job I had been given fairer treatment than on any previous job and *not* for personal reasons nor had it been tied up in any way with my brief personal relationship with Mr. X, who was part of the firm."

One day, on impulse, I went to her office and demanded that she quit her job on the spot. She did. It was a very great humiliation for her.

And then, despite my agreement that we both live by a single standard, I returned to my New School flirtations and after-work dates.

It was for her, I think, the cruelest time period of our entire married life.

"This was not a repressed suffering that Lyle knew nothing of," she wrote. "He knew in everything I said and did. . . . It was very quickly apparent to him that I would do anything he wanted, that I did not want other men, that I would never have a personal relationship with another man again because I wanted only Lyle and I wanted only that our life together should be good."

Eventually I grew up—at least a little. . . .

It isn't possible to telescope all the many excitements of our lives together. We came to know and to love a circle of friends. Dick and Lil Manning. Leonard and Eleanor Green. Joe Whalen. Avant Keels. There were occasional dull hours but never a dull day.

I quit my job at the ready-to-wear paper when the owner fired a girl for coming to work ten minutes late. I decided to free-lance because it would allow Mary Louise and me to be together again as we had been during the happy days I wrote my novel.

Our lease in Hell's Kitchen had run out. We rented a new garden-type apartment in North Bergen, New Jersey.

I wrote our way to food and shelter. Comic strip continuities for John Wayne comics and Billy the Kid. Scripts for the State Department's Voice of America. Scripts for the American Medical Association. Columns (ghosted) for Walter Winchell.

And then, one day late in 1951, with slightly more than $1,000 to our names and next month's rent coming due, we decided to launch the paper Exposé—now known as The Independent.

That story has been told in the pages of *The Independent* many times. But never with small details like this:

Subscriptions came in. We didn't know anything about handling subscriptions. How do you record them? How do you control expiration dates?

Mary Louise spent a few days thinking about it. And then she created our subscription system. It is still used without variation today.

Someone had to keep books and records. We knew nothing about bookkeeping or accounting.

Mary Louise bought a book on the subject for $1.95. She studied it and set up a bookkeeping system. She had known not a thing about keeping books. But years later, when a top C.P.A. came to examine the books, he marveled at the sophisticated perfection of the system. He could suggest no improvements.

She was that way in everything she did. Calm, resolute, incredibly competent.

She was genuine, perhaps too much so for New York. She took people at their word—and forgave them when they broke it.

One afternoon, we attended a broadcast at WCBS. It was the coast-to-coast Landt Trio "Sing Along" program. I had once managed the Landts, and Mary Louise had come to know and like them.

Carl Landt spotted us immediately. He began to select people for his little quiz in which the audience members were invited to the stage for a chance to win silver dollars answering typically simple-minded radio quiz questions.

"Let's have that lovely redhead in the balcony," he said, pointing up to her.

Reluctantly, she went down to the studio stage.

"And what is your name, beautiful lady?" Carl asked.

"Why Carl, you know me!" she said, perplexed.

Coast to coast.

The Landt Trio and CBS were never quite the same after that.

She was always immaculate. Flawless. Delightful to look at and a pleasure to be with.

She was critical of fashion design. She wore thonged sandals and form-fitting slacks many years before they became the thing to wear. And she was immensely fond of simple hanging earrings.

But she never developed any desire for expensive jewelry. Except for some handsome Monet costume pieces given to her by our friends, the Mannings, she rarely wore anything that cost more than a few dollars.

Three years ago, when we were in Rio de Janeiro, I saw and bought for her the most beautiful flexible gold necklace, set with sparkling diamonds and blue sapphires. It was a work of art. I paid $3,000 for it.

She loved the necklace for its contemporary design, fine workmanship, and startlingly simple beauty. But she never wore it. Not once. Occasionally, when I pressed her about it, she said she was looking for a simple black velvet dress that it would go with. The simple things didn't seem to be around and it appeared that she would have to design and make her own.

Ostentation was simply not her style.

She loved Rory and Sandy. Rory was born in natural childbirth. We located the only hospital in the entire city that allowed complete rooming-in. Only four beds were so allocated. From the moment he was born, he was at her side in his crib and she was taking full care of him. She was a nursing mother, of course. And, of course, we did not permit the doctors to circumcise him.

There would have been no *Independent* without her. She had an acute sense for the precise word to use and a balanced attitude toward the most controversial subjects. She tempered my editorials. She was the only censor I ever respected.

With no more than two or three exceptions, she proofread, in entirety, every issue of *The Independent* for nearly eighteen years.

When, this spring, it was impossible to burden her with the proofreading, I simply stopped producing the paper. The "April" issue which recently went into the mail was totally produced by a guest editor.

There would have been no book publishing venture without her. Over and over again the books that really counted went into production because she said they should.

I cite, as a single example of what I mean, the case of Ferdinand Lundberg. When Professor Lundberg and I discussed the possibility of his researching and writing a book about who controls America today, he explained that he would have to have living expenses for two and one-half years. Paying a substantial advance of this kind was totally alien to our policy.

But when I happened to mention the Lundberg conversation to Mary Louise, she responded simply: "You have to publish that book. Whatever it may cost and whatever money you lose on it, publish it. You have a moral responsibility to publish it."

The Rich and the Super-Rich became the most profitable book we published up to that time.

One morning, on my birthday, I left her in bed sleeping and quietly headed for New York. A short distance from my door I was attacked by three hired thugs with blackjacks.

By my next birthday, we had moved to an apartment in Greenwich Village. When I awoke, there was a note next to the bed.

"Good morning," it said. "Happy birthday! I love you. Please don't go out without me."

One day I wrote her a very long prose poem. It began,

I can not truly tell you
What you mean to me
Because words are inadequate
And impersonal

Because you use a word
And it has been used before
In different times, in different places
In different ways
Until its meaning has been sapped from it
By the popular love songs
And the slogans in the subways
And the multiple myths
Upon myths upon myths upon myths
In movies and plays and books
And poems.
To tell you that I love you
More than anything else in the world
More, I think, than life itself

May perhaps sound corny.
Words strung together as they have
*   been strung together since words began*
Inadequate
Impersonal.
To tell you that I love you
Beyond any love I have ever felt
For anyone
Even myself
Is no sonnet
And not very original
And yet my love for you
Seems so beyond what ordinary men
Must feel about ordinary women.
How can I tell you?

And many pages later,

I have, as you know, a kind of a sense of destiny,
fleeting time, so little time, and death. The
days pass, the years pass, and the final sleep, the
last sleep, draws nearer
And it does not matter: we do not matter
Except to each other
It is difficult to say, and yet it must be said
Somehow, however poorly.
How,
The times I feel myself most aware
of the slow turn of time
Of the people who will be sitting here

a hundred years from tonight
Unaware of our having ever lived
Or lived to gather together
Some precious happiness . . .
Those times are most often in the early morn-
   ing hours.
And I worry then. Morbid. Depressed. While
   most of
our world and the people we know are sleeping.
   While
you are sleeping.
I worry because I know that it is inevitable that
someday we will not be together.
In death it would not matter to me. In life
   I would be
lost without you.

I became business manager of Bill Gaines' magazines and helped to turn *Mad* from a ten-cent
comic book to a 25¢ magazine.

Then, unintentionally, I had backed into book
publishing, using, as my capital, money I had collected in a libel action against Walter Winchell
and *Confidential*.

Sandy was nearly thirteen and Rory nearly four
when we began to travel. We started with 21 days
in Europe in 1960. Every year after that we went
to Europe at least once and sometimes twice.

Frankfurt, for the book fair. London. Enchanting Copenhagen. Oslo. Prague. Belgrade. Paris (which we didn't like). Rome (which we loved).

There were Puerto Rico and Acapulco and Los Angeles and San Francisco. There were Rio de Janeiro and Monte Carlo and Freeport and Bermuda and Ocho Rios and Las Vegas.

Eventually, as I could afford it, I became a "high roller" in the casinos. I enjoyed casino gambling, and she learned to enjoy it too.

We visited Cuba three times after the Revolution. Once with both children and once with only my son.

She learned to play craps in Havana. She was so genuinely sweet that the stick men and the box men could not help but like her.

We were at a reception given by Dr. Fidel Castro at the Presidential Palace when he learned that the United States had broken relations with Cuba.

Many Americans panicked. They made desperate phone calls to the States. They flocked to the American Embassy. They talked about getting to Guantanamo.

We returned to the Havana Riviera and went to the casino. It was very busy, but very quiet. We began to throw the dice. Finally, I remarked: "Do you know that the U.S. has broken relations with Cuba?"

The men at the table smiled. "We know," they

assured me. "But that does not mean that we must break relations with you."

We won that night. And with the pesos, she bought a collection of Portocarrero original paintings. Our friend, Edmundo Desnoes, took her to the artist's home.

I have gambled in many parts of the world. I've had gamblers' lucky streaks and I've had losers. On balance, I have lost a substantial amount of money—but never anything that would jeopardize us.

She, on the other hand, played for much smaller stakes—and she invariably won. She was an amazing gambler. She enjoyed every minute of it, but she was always under complete control. If anything at all bothered her at a blackjack or craps table, she left immediately. It could be a cigar or the voice of a dealer or the lack of ventilation. Anything.

She won so consistently because she knew just what she was doing. As she explained it: "Almost every time you gamble, there is a period where you are ahead. Most people continue to play until they lose. My philosophy is to quit when you're ahead."

On one occasion I lost more money than I would care to record here. She used to try to guess from the expression on my face whether I was a winner or a loser. And I would try to fool her. It was our game. This time, there was no game. It must have been written all over my face.

She took my hand and we walked out of the casino into the garden.

"Have you lost a lot of money?" she asked.

"A big amount."

"Perhaps we should take a rest from Las Vegas," she suggested. "How bad was it?"

"Pretty bad." I told her the figure.

"That *is* a lot of money," she said. "Do you love me?" she asked.

"More than anything in the world."

"Well, that's how I love you—so we haven't really lost anything, have we?"

I don't know any other wives like that.

She enjoyed being with me in Vegas. We both knew that the royal treatment we received—the penthouse suites and the free food and drink and front-row seats at the shows in every major hotel on the strip—was all part of the game they played.

It was in Las Vegas on our first trip there that we met Bonnie and Mickey Leffert. He was a subscriber to *The Independent*. We came to have such high regard for both of them that, unbeknownst to them, we wrote our wills so that, if something were to happen to the both of us, they were to be asked to raise our two children.

Gambling was my luxury. She finally found one of her own to indulge in.

It happened this way. We had bought a piece of land in Jamaica, sight unseen. We bought it from an artist who had once been wealthy but had since run into financial reverses.

We visited Jamaica for the first time two years later.

"It's lovely," I said, struggling through the dense bush. "Now let's put it on the market and get rid of it."

"Don't sell it," she said.

"Don't sell it, daddy," our little boy echoed.

"Someday we ought to build a house here," she said.

She began to plan the house three years ago. She was her own designer: we hired no architect. Her friend, Faye Fingesten, helped her select furniture.

After many frustrating delays, construction began in October, 1968. The house had developed into something of a mansion. The building contract called for completion within eight months.

In addition to the main house, there would be a guest house that could hold eight and a staff house and a large swimming pool.

We conduct an unusual business. Once very year or so, our offices are closed and the entire staff is taken on a journey. We spend ten days to three weeks going to a new foreign place. The time is mostly "bonus" vacation time for the employees—and all expenses are paid. Everyone lives like a millionaire. We stay at the very finest hotels, eat the very finest food, hire our own fleet of automobiles and, when we visit a gaming casino, everyone is given gambling money.

Actually it has turned out to be an excellent business policy though it was never intended that way. Our office staff is like one large family.

My secretary, Carole Livingston, recently observed that for a long time she hadn't realized the important role that Mary Louise played in things like the bonus office trips. And then she began to become aware that Mary Louise was the key to them. For it was Mary Louise who was acutely opposed to exploiting people and who wanted everyone to have the best things in life.

We took the office staff to San Juan. Later, to Acapulco. Later to Ocho Rios, Jamaica. Then, last year, we decided to treat everybody to a 22-day all-expense tour of the cities in Europe that we had come to know and like: London, Copenhagen, Monte Carlo, and Rome.

Some nightmares begin on sunny days in bright sunny places. They begin in small ways with small things that one doesn't notice.

*At the train depot
in Orange Heights, Florida*

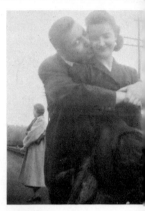

*On the street in
Akron, Ohio, 1945*

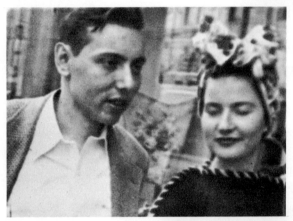

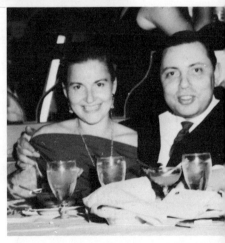

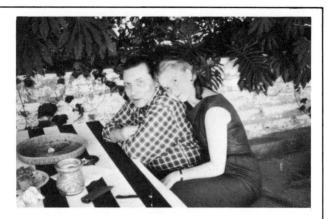

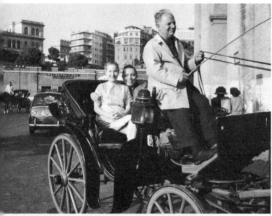

Rome, 1967

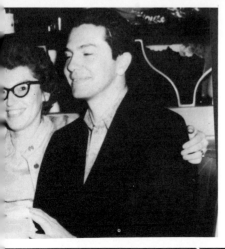

Havana, 1960:
Mary Louise and Lyle Stuart
with Irma and
Irving Greenbaum

Take the hamsters. One day I passed a pet shop and saw some baby hamsters. I brought home a collection of them. They multiplied. I enjoyed them. We kept them in the living room.

A couple of weeks later, she began to itch. She took hot showers. The itch continued and became more uncomfortable. It reached the point where she couldn't sleep at night for more than a couple of hours at a time without bathing.

I didn't connect it with the hamsters. And then one day I lay on the living room couch watching a television program, and I began to itch.

We gave away the hamsters within twenty-four hours. We both stopped itching within another twenty-four. She and I had both, obviously, reacted to the hamster dander. She also spoke of a digestive complaint. To this day I keep telling myself that none of it could have caused what followed—but I can never be sure.

Digestive complaints came and went. She wasn't feeling up to her usual self. I suggested that we postpone the office tour of Europe, but she would hear no more of that.

We went. She concealed her pain. She would not spoil anyone's pleasure.

In December, we went to Las Vegas. Friends expressed concern that her "stomach ache" was lasting too long.

For many months she had tried to treat herself with diet control. A week on nothing but grape juice. A week on tuna fish and grapes. At times, things seemed to improve.

At the suggestion that she might be suffering a tropical disease, we sought out the number one man in that field. His report: negative.

She couldn't stabilize her pulse. She didn't tell me. There was blood in her stool. She didn't tell me.

In January, we made a hurried journey to Jamaica to observe the progress of the house. We went there only after she promised me that, on our return, she would submit to a complete physical examination at Life Extension Institute.

The examination was scheduled for Tuesday morning. On Monday night she was restless and couldn't sleep. At 2 a.m. she sat up and I was instantly alert.

"What is it, sweetie?"

"I feel foolish," she said. "I'm worried."

"About what?"

"The staff quarters. Do you think the staff house is far enough away from the main house not to seem to be crowding it? Would it be too late to change it?"

My anxiety about her health made me angry. "For heaven's sake, sweetie, let's forget about the house in Jamaica and worry instead about getting you completely well again!"

She didn't reply and her silence spoke volumes.

"Okay," I said, quieting down. "It will probably cost a fortune to move the staff house now, but if that's what you want, that's what we'll do."

She smiled and kissed me. "Maybe it isn't too close," she said. "We'll let it stay where it is."

The nightmare accelerated the next day.

The arrangement was that she could go for the examination while I consulted with our attorney, Jack Albert. We'd meet at noon on the second floor of the Mercantile Library on 47th Street off Madison Avenue.

I was delayed. When I walked into the library she was coming down the stairs from the second floor. She was smiling and I felt a quick surge of relief.

"Are you okay?" I asked.

She took my hand. "Let's go upstairs," she said. "I have to talk with you."

We walked up the stairs and sat down at one of the tables. She was still smiling.

"The doctor said I have a growth in my lower colon. He says I should have a biopsy right away."

The room blackened. She was consoling me. "I'm sorry, sweetheart," she said, "but don't worry yet. It may not be anything."

"Where do we go?" I asked.

"They aren't supposed to suggest specific doctors but he gave me the card of a man who was his instructor in medical school."

"Let's get to him right away," I said.

"Let's."

Try to find a public telephone in midtown Manhattan. One after the other: out of order. At last we found a group of phones in a cigar store, surrounded by a cluster of people waiting to use them. She pressed my hand as we waited an eternity for one to be available for us.

The doctor was in Hawaii. He wouldn't return until Monday. That was a week away.

I remembered a surgeon who had performed some minor surgery on me. We taxied to his office. He had gone for the day but his receptionist was able to summon him to return.

After an examination, the surgeon told me: "I'm ninety percent sure it's malignant."

Tears and hysteria. Mine, not hers. She was gentle. Reassuring me that it wasn't all that bad.

The nightmare accelerated.

She had some very firm ideas about what was to come. If it was cancer and if it had spread, she did not want to be carved up.

"A person has the right to choose what she wants to do," she insisted.

She was also firm against a colostomy. She was too fastidious.

"See here," the surgeon said, "if it will save your life to give you a temporary colostomy—just for a few weeks—I'm going to do it."

She was still concerned that he would carve her up. I assured her that he wouldn't. I told him (he became indignant) that, if he opened her abdomen and found it had spread, he was to sew her up again and I would pay a fee equal to what he'd charge if he had performed the cutting up.

I described the operation in the January issue of *The Independent*.

In the February issue, I reported that, "She has completely recovered from the effects of the operation. She has put on weight and is more beautiful than ever. . . ."

It was the truth, but it was an incomplete report.

This is what I didn't report.

While she was in the recovery room, the surgeon returned to her private room in Doctors Hospital, where I had been pacing the floor for nearly four hours.

He told me that she would be all right "for now" and that he hadn't given her a colostomy.

And then he pronounced her death sentence. He had found three large nodules on the right lobe of her liver.

He became a philosopher, trying to console me.

"We are all doing to die," he said. "What this means is that the probability is she'll die of tumor of the liver. That is, if Mack's Truck disease doesn't get her first. I mean, if she isn't hit by a truck on the street or something like that. . . .

"She may live for many years. She may outlive you."

"I want to give you some advice," he added. "And listen very carefully to me. I know how fond you are of each other and how honest you are with each other. But you absolutely must not tell her what I've told you. No matter how you think she'd accept it, you mustn't tell. I've had thirty years of experience and I know what I'm talking about. If you tell her, she'll turn against you and she'll turn against her own children."

"I can't lie to her."

"You must."

For a moment I recalled an incident that had occurred on the previous day. She'd been in the X-ray room. They had kept her waiting a long time in a wheel chair. And then she fainted riding down the hospital elevator.

They wheeled her into her room and began to revive her.

She told me later in the day: "You know, as I was regaining consciousness I felt a terrible panic and wanted to get up from the chair and run away. And then I saw you standing there and I knew I was safe."

Would she know she was safe when she saw my face after the operation? After never lying to her about any serious matter, could I conceal the horror of my knowledge from my face?

I tried. For her sake, I tried. Desperately. I succeeded.

I was in the room sixteen hours a day or more. In a few days she began to recover. The surgeon visited her.

"You should have come to me sooner," he said.

"Why?" she said cheerfully. "What's the difference? You said you got it all, didn't you?"

He nodded.

I had to tell someone. I told Bill Gaines and Dick and Lil Manning. And then I began to think that I was going to lose my mind.

I phoned Dr. Albert Ellis. "Al, I have to see you. Right away. Professionally."

It was my first visit to a psychologist. He listened. And then he told me: "The doctor is right about most people. Most people can't take it. But Mary Louise is the one in a hundred who could. If you feel your way and she seems to want to know, by all means tell her."

She had returned to our apartment in Brooklyn and was in bed when I told her.

I was lying in the bed beside her. "I have to tell you something," I said. "Sweetheart, I don't want to. I have been going half out of my mind. But I have never lied to you about anything important and I can't lie to you now."

We held hands and I told her.

"You were right in telling me," she said. "Of course you were right in telling me."

She lay still for ten minutes staring at the ceiling. "Since you say there's nothing we can do about it, let's talk about other things."

Later she said: "I wish you wouldn't worry. It will depress me terribly to see you depressed. Look, sweetie, I've had a little while to think. I couldn't have taken this a year ago because Rory was too dependent on me. But he is weaned now. He has his own friends and he's growing up fast. He's his own young man and he's going to be a fine young man."

She continued: "Sandy is nearly twenty-two. She has turned out to be a delight too. She's making some mistakes but she'll find herself. It's you I'm worried about."

And later: "Do you know something crazy? I don't think I believed how much you really cared about me until you cried that day in the doctor's office."

She continued to make plans for the house in Jamaica.

A few weeks later she had seemingly recovered.

She gained weight. She went about her daily chores as if nothing had happened to change anything.

In February we threw a party for fifty people. She was her cheerful self. Only she and I and three of the guests knew.

"We mustn't tell the children," she said. "Not now, anyway. It would spoil too many things for them."

A few evenings after I told her, she phoned her surgeon. They had become fast telephone friends. Our family had been to his home and his family to ours.

At the end of this conversation, she said in her cute way: "Oh, doctor, there's one more thing. I want you to promise not to lie to me again. I want to be able to believe what you tell me."

"What are you talking about?" he said.

"I'll give you two words. Liver involvement."

He seemed stunned. When he could recover he could only say, "Your husband is an idiot."

"Never mind," she said. "Just don't lie to me in the future."

Someone I considered a friend wrote to me: "The philosophy of medicine which we consider to be the most comprehensive, the most profound, the most logical, benign and beneficial involves the *total* approach to the patient. It embraces all deficiencies (such as pancreas, spleen, liver, etc.) to mention a few metabolic conditions. In other words, instead of fractionating the patient by pinpointing one small area of his body and concentrating the therapy on that point, it rallies *all* the forces of the body to meet the challenge of the disease . . . for cancer is a *systemic* disease. The entire system must therefore be supported so that it may reconstitute itself and permit the cells to return to normal." The friend recommended a doctor.

Thus did we have our experience with quackery.

The doctor involved was an M.D. She was a messianic quack. She feels that it is her mission in life to cure cancer. She is self-duped. The pathetic thing is that she is honest. She isn't out to swindle anyone. True, she feels the medical association hounds her, but otherwise she seems rational and scientific.

Mary Louise visited her once a week. But the "treatment" began to bother me. The doctor never gave her a physical examination. There were blood tests and high-sounding medical proclamations. There were various pills of many sizes and colors.

The liver tumor began to grow. Mary Louise could feel it.

Now the quack doctor had a new suggestion. Why didn't we try Krebiozen? She had some of the *original* issue. She would be happy to give it to Mary Louise.

The original Krebiozen had long ago lost its effectiveness so that, toward the end, patients were receiving ten times the normal dose. On top of that, the *original* was contained in mineral oil that left lumps wherever it was injected.

Dr. Quack explained: "You get one injection and then another 72 hours later and then another one week later."

That hasn't been the approach in nearly five years! The substance is given twice a day for a week and thereafter once a day.

I was sick to my stomach when I realized how deluded and irresponsible Dr. Quack was. And she was toying with human lives.

I read. I consulted with the so-called "top men" in the field. I researched. According to the Lahey Clinic, she could expect to survive anywhere from one month to four years. But of 41 patients, only seven lived as long as two years.

"Give her 5-FU," I was advised.

I read all the literature on Fluorouracil. Then I faced one of the world's foremost specialists, and listened as he told me to try 5-FU.

"If 5-FU works, why isn't it used *before* surgery?" I inquired.

It was as if I had struck him on the jaw with my fist. He said in a weak voice, "Well, you're right, you know. We used to use it before surgery but now we no longer do."

"Then how in the world can anybody say that it is any good after surgery?"

He went to his files and handed me a paper. It was a speech he'd read at a medical meeting a year before. "Sometimes," he had said, "the best thing to do is to do nothing."

I was not willing to do nothing.

I heard 5-FU until it was coming out of my ears. Phony claims. Phony statistics. The toxic side effects spelled out. But nowhere the clear statement that while 5-FU destroys "bad" cells it always destroys good ones—and thus is a death sentence in and of itself.

Mary Louise began to show signs of fatigue. She was concerned about buying furniture for the Jamaica house. We flew to Denmark for the Easter weekend. We didn't know that Thursday, Friday, Sunday, and Monday would all be legal holidays with all the stores closed.

She had Saturday in which to make all of her purchases—and the stores closed at 2 p.m. We bought a few things at Den Permanente. Mostly, however, we bought at Illums Bolighus, and the manager showed her special attention, leading her through the warehouse and remaining with her until long after the store had closed to the public.

Rory John was with us. We flew to Interlaken so he could ski. We took the scenic train ride to Kleine Scheidegg. Mary Louise rented skis for herself too. She made her way up the busy slope to a class where the instructor said she could join his group. But then he became too busy to show her how to properly fasten her skis, so she returned. She was exhausted, but obviously pleased about Rory's happy ski adventuring. Too, she enjoyed the beautiful Swiss mountainside.

She rested a great deal, but she was still quite able to walk. Sometimes it seemed to the both of us as though our fears were all fanciful and that she was just tired and would relax and soon be her old self again.

"If a person can will themselves to stay well," she said, "then I'm doing it."

In May, she and I flew to Jamaica. As usual, we stayed at the Playboy. It's near our property—being about eight miles away—and the staff knew us and always treated us with special courtesy.

It was while she was unpacking that she reached into her pocketbook and took out a letter I had written to her exactly ten years earlier.

Dated May 7, 1959, it began:

"Dear Mary Louise,

"I love you. I truly and honestly do.

"In reflecting on things, it is interesting to re-

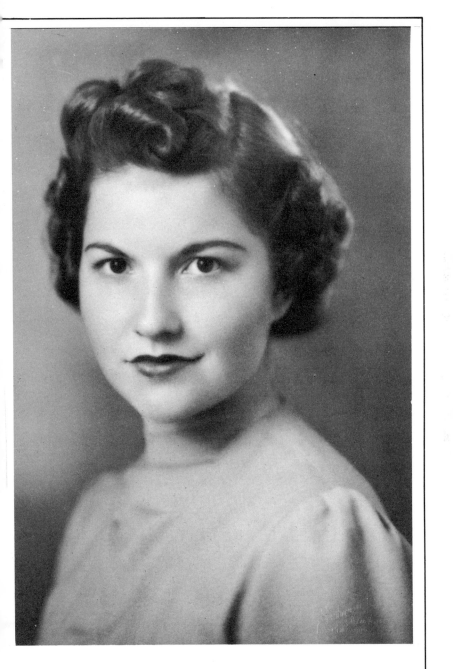

call how my feelings about so many people and attitudes have changed through the years. For example, do you recall my 'politics' when first we met? Or my attitudes toward money, mother, aunts etc., clothes, life spans, and so many of the other objects toward which I've changed my views and emotions?

"And yet, despite everything (and there have been many things) my love for you has remained constant, abiding, stronger thru the years.

"You are my everything. Without you I am nothing.

"These are not just 'words.' They are the very essence of what reality there is to my whole life. . . ."

I held the letter out. "What are you doing with this?"

She sat on the bed, looking at me with love in her eyes.

"I just happened to come upon it the other day," she said. "Read the last page."

"Beneath the outer trappings," I had written, "we all live in our separate worlds with our secret dreams, self-images, and sweet sorrows. We are strangers when we meet and strangers when we marry, and when you think about it all, when you think about two strangers from separate worlds and with their own separate inner worlds, and these two strangers meet and are drawn together by self-love and selfish love and whatever it is that draws one man to one woman and one woman to one man—and fills them with the naïve belief that they can join in a marriage ritual and then live happily ever after—when you think about it, you can't be astounded that so many strangers go their separate ways after a year or two or the statistical three.

"And then when you think about the millions who stay together because that's what people do or religions say to do or for want of any other place to be or things to do . . . and how few care much about the other and how many are trapped and know not where to find the key. . . .

"When you think about these things and how they are the way the humans are and the way the humans do . . . and you think about how rare it is for a husband to love his wife one year later as he did on the morning of the first evening he would make love to her. . . .

"And then you think about our trials and tribulations (but never any genuine doubt that we will stay together and be together)—and then the four of us who used to be two, complicating our lives, multiplying our problems—and thru it all, the days and weeks and years—and with our shortcomings (my many, your few)—and the sultry wiggle of circumstance—and when you realize that thru it all my love for you has grown, my lust for you, my longing for you, my fondness for you—all fresh and alive and young—it hasn't been bad from my side.

"But for you, I don't think I would have ever known what it was to really love. All the happiness I have ever known I have known because of you. I have told you these things years ago in letters.

"I wish that I had been able to provide you with more of a share of happiness and contentment than I have. But our lives together are not over. With a little bit of luck, they are scarcely begun. And the world is new and the scraps of the past are fluttering around us and you're coming down High Street toward me and already, without understanding how it happened, you have enchanted me—as you have rarely since then stopped enchanting me—and the music I hear goes with a portrait of a little boy lost who is about to find himself in a warm, tender vision—and saying the words to himself 'I love her, I love her, I love her.'

"And I have never stopped saying those words, my beloved. And I never shall.

"I love Mary Louise. I love Mary Louise. I love you."

I returned the letter to her.

"You really don't need this," I said lightly. "You've got me."

"Please don't ever stop loving me," she said. "I know I may become a big problem to you, but please don't ever stop loving me. I don't know what I'd do if you ever stopped loving me."

Again, Lady Circumstance took a hand in the proceedings.

Our plan had been to retire early and in the morning to visit the property and begin the rounds with builder, solicitor (lawyer), and the others. Now we looked at each other and I looked at my watch. It was only 4:30 p.m.

"What do you say we take a quick ride to see how much they've done?" I asked.

"Let's."

"You're not too tired?"

"No."

I wasn't pleased by what we saw. The construction seemed to be taking forever. We would have plenty to say to the builder on the morrow. And then, we walked toward our car to leave when an air-conditioned Oldsmobile drove up the road. It contained two women.

"What are they doing on our land?" I asked our foreman, in a voice loud enough for them to hear.

The woman at the wheel was flustered. She hastily introduced herself as Blanche Blackwell and apologized for trespassing. She was a lively, vivacious woman in her early fifties and I was surprised. I had heard of Mrs. Blackwell and had imagined her a seventy-year-old crotchety dame who leaned on a cane and sat in her famed mansion barking orders and counting her money.

Noel Coward was our nearest white neighbor. He had a place on top of the mountain at the end of the road that led past our property. He had a guest house on the road facing the ocean. Both properties had been bought from Blanche Blackwell.

Ian Fleming had written his thirteen James Bond books at Golden Eye in Oracabessa. His lovely Golden Eye estate and beach, next to the banana boat wharf, were leased to Blanche Blackwell.

Our own land, bought from our artist friend, had been a part of the Wentworth Estate. It and thousands of additional acres that contained banana plantations and coconut plantations and a copra factory and a cattle herd and a riding stable were all owned by Blanche Blackwell.

Her home, the famous Bolt House, had been the dining place for so many of the visiting celebrities to the island. Anthony Eden and Ralph Bunche and Oona O'Neill Chaplin and dozens and dozens of others.

Errol Flynn in his autobiography *My Wicked,*

Wicked Ways described his first visit to Blanche Blackwell's Bolt House: "Never had I seen a land so beautiful. Now I knew where the writers of the Bible had gotten their description of paradise. They had come here to Jamaica and then their words had been set down and they have been read ever since."

Flynn also wrote of Blanche Blackwell: "I arrived and met this pale-faced girl with the dark, intense eyes and beautiful teeth, and a laugh like the sound of water tinkling over a waterfall. We fell into the most animated conversation. I had come from one end of the earth and she lived here, at the other, and yet it seemed that we had whole worlds to speak of. . . .

"I can only say for Blanche Blackwell, who not long afterwards was divorced from Joe, that she and I became the fastest friends to the point where I thought of proposing—while still married to Nora—but I feared a rejection and perhaps a difference in our relationship. Blanche and I formed an enduring friendship amazingly platonic."

Flynn also wrote: "This would be my base forever, two or three months a year, or five months a year. It reminded me of all the beauty of the Polynesian Islands . . . all around was the sea, fine tropic foods, rare sea foods . . . and sun, wonderful year-round sun. After thirty-seven years of wandering I had found my Grecian isle."

Blanche Blackwell explained that she had come here often "curious and fascinated by knowing that anyone is doing what you're doing in a place like this."

She invited us to tea at Bolt House but said that we would have to visit in the morning. It seems that she was preparing to leave Bolt House in the afternoon for an itinerary that might take as long as five years.

Had we not driven to our place that evening, we might never have met her.

How very lucky we were, that evening. . . .

We had a tight schedule the next day. And in the morning when I had checked the car out of Hertz and come out of the Playboy, I found Mary Louise sitting on the steps, obviously ill. She couldn't go. Why didn't I go myself to see all those people we had to see? I told her that was a foolish suggestion and led her back to our room. She upchucked and immediately felt better.

We visited our place again. And then, on the way to Ocho Rios, stopped off at Bolt House.

Bolt is a truly lovely place. Spacious, open, thoroughly comfortable. It has a pink and white decor. It was fourteen years old and Blanche Blackwell had done the unusual thing of having an American architect brought to the island to direct its construction.

A man entered, kissed her. "Ah ha!" I thought. "Her lover!" But then, as they conversed, it turned out that he had four children and she thought he had two. No lover. He was, in fact, Ian Pringle, a member of Lord Ronald Graham's organization. He had come to talk with her about the Graham organization renting Bolt occasionally during her absence.

I did some quick calculating. Although our contractor had assured me our guest house would be finished, it was doubtful if the main house would be done by July 1—which was when we planned to return to Jamaica. That meant that Mary Louise would be subject to all the building noises.

I gingerly asked if Mrs. Blackwell would object to renting her house to us. We would be its first rental tenants. Blanche Blackwell was startled. She was so involved with her house that she was fearful of letting unknown strangers occupy it and she would be very relaxed if we were the first renters.

She conferred with Pringle about price while Mary Louise and I walked through the lovely gardens and looked at the pool. A maid explained that the donkey on the lawn and the funny little car in the driveway belonged to rock and roll singer Tommy Steele and were being kept for him as a favor.

By now I knew I would pay *any* price for Mary

Louise to have the comfort the house promised. I was surprised at how reasonable a price was being asked. I surprised them in turn by immediately paying for the month of July in full.

Even now I dread to imagine what July and August would have been like if we hadn't gone to the Stuart place that night and met Blanche Blackwell and through the accidental meeting, rented Bolt House. . . .

The liver pains began a few days after our return from Jamaica. Mary Louise stayed in bed.

Her surgeon said he could do nothing: there was nothing he could do. He prescribed a mild narcotic syrup to ease the pain but it had no effect.

I began to make plans for securing Krebiozen (now called "Carcalon") and at the same time I searched my mind for any alternatives. Was there somebody, somewhere, who had discovered something that had not yet gotten out of a research laboratory? How to locate it? A way suggested itself to me. I wrote an ad for the *New York Times*.

The *Times* turned it down. It had been submitted to the local medical society and had been disapproved because I was, in theory at least, inviting nonmedical people to practice medicine.

I became frantic. I appealed to Harding Bancroft, Executive Vice President of the *Times*. He passed the buck to Vice President Ivan Veit. Veit phoned me and asked the purpose of the ad. I explained it to him.

"I'm going to overrule the censor and the medical board," he said finally. "You have every right to try everything you can to help your wife."

Love that Ivan Veit.

The ad ran. It looked like this:

$25,000 REWARD

My wife has hepatic metastases (cancer of the liver). I will pay $25,000 to any person (physician, surgeon, chemist, etc.) who can keep her alive and ambulatory for one year. Approach must be sound and logical.   Box V 112 TIMES

It was to run in the Public Notice section, which faces the television page, and thus could be widely read. On the day it appeared, however, a TV network decided to run a full page facing the TV page, so the public-notice column was pushed forward. I quickly ordered another insertion for two days later. Again a TV network took the full page.

I waited.

We did something then that has probably since saved my sanity. Each afternoon, when she was up to it, I tape-recorded conversation with Mary Louise.

Our talks were cheerful, sprinkled with her laughter. She recollected her days on the farm and then we both remembered our early meetings and the days and years of our being together.

There were nearly five hours of conversation. And then we made a tape on which I asked her what to do about various problems which might arise.

The ads in the *Times* brought more than 450 responses. Bill Gaines helped me evaluate them. And by the time we were through, I knew that I had touched all bases.

The responses broke down this way. There were a hundred or so full of religious nonsense. There were holy cards from priests and nuns and religious pamphlets and booklets and prayers. They were pitiful. And I was surprised that people like that were *Times* rather than *News* readers.

There were forty letters in Spanish and in Norwegian—for the story had been picked up by Spanish newspapers and by one in Norway.

There were a hundred or so letters from surgeons, physicians, biochemists, radiologists.

Let me tell you about two of them. It is sadly ironic what an offer of $25,000 can do.

There was one cancer specialist in New York with whom I had spoken by phone. A friend of mine had once paid about $1,000 to translate some material from Japanese on an anti-cancer substance being tested in Japan. I wanted the material. If the specialist couldn't locate it, I would pay the $1,000 again to have it translated.

He promised to look for it and let me know "one way or the other within a couple of days."

I phoned him four times. Twice a week for two weeks. I never got through to him—only to his secretary. And each time I asked only for a "yes" or "no" regarding the material. I didn't get it and gave up.

He was too busy. But he wasn't too busy to send a two-page 8½-x-11 typewritten letter to the anonymous person who offered the $25,000 reward.

Another of the interesting examples involved the surgeon who had been successful with liver transplant operations. I had tried desperately to get through to him but his receptionist had firmly explained that he was too occupied and it was doubtful in a case such as Mary Louise's that he would consider a transplant. Now, he wrote to me too. . . .

The press responded to the anonymous ad, of course. NBC and CBS. The Associated Press and World Wide Features. Reuters. A reporter and an editor from *Life* magazine. News Limited of Australia.

There was a particularly callous reply from a drippy-sounding woman at *The News* who identified herself as Linda Scarbrough, "science editor," and who thought "it would make a fine special feature to see the cross-section of people your advertisement attracts."

There were also some very sweet, encouraging letters. And there were some very helpful ones. Outstanding in its comprehensiveness was one from Elaine Swenson of the Society for Language Research.

After selecting eight letters that seemed worth following up, I mimeographed a "thank you" note which was sent to all the others. It said in part:

"You are one of the many hundreds of men and women kind enough to take the time and trouble to write to me. My wife and I want to thank you for this. I am sorry that the intensity of my problem and the large number of letters received makes it impossible to answer all of them personally. . . .

". . . To the variety of newspapers and magazines who offered to do stories: I appreciate your interest but no, thanks. My wife's illness is not a circus and we are not interested in publicity. . . .

". . . To those people who sent us religious tracts, holy pictures and other such nonsense. Both my wife and I appreciate the goodwill that moved these people to respond . . . [but] my wife and I are rational thinkers. We consider most religion insanity—and all belief in any personal god or gods to be total foolishness. We are not 'agnostics'—

we are atheists. Our lovely children—bright and wholesome—are also atheists. That anyone could believe that a 'holy picture' or some collection of words mumbled over and over compulsively could change the course of nature is a rather pathetic commentary on the current state of mankind. We hope that in our children's time, men and women will be courageous and sensible enough to throw off all the shackles of fear, compulsion and superstition that make the religious rackets so profitable. . . .

"My wife and I are in our forties. We have been married 23 years. We are very much in love with each other.

"In recent years—as an almost accidental side effect rather than as a goal—I have made a considerable amount of money. I set the reward at $25,000—but could have made it $100,000 . . . and would, indeed, give every material thing I own to bring my wife back to good health. . . ."

A few days later at the *Times* box, there was a very sweet letter from one of the editors of *Life*. He loved his wife too and knew how I felt.

The supply of Carcalon (Krebiozen) is limited. It cannot be shipped interstate.

I phoned Mary Louise's surgeon. "Dr. L., I'm flying to Chicago for some of this substance. I've pulled a few strings and it is being made available to me. I'm going to want you to show me how to inject it. Also, there's something called the linear accelerator that I want to try."

"I'll do anything I can to help you," he said.

I didn't know then that this medical worm had already lied to Mary Louise and had told her he had "tried Krebiozen on six or seven patients and it didn't do any good."

I didn't learn it until that evening when I returned from Chicago. I had met Dr. Andrew Ivy again and he had shown me his laboratory. I made an unsolicited contribution to his research.

Dr. L. phoned me before I could call him. He wanted to meet with me that evening, but I was too exhausted. My daughter, Sandra Lee, had come to Chicago from the University of Wisconsin at Madison to spend a few hours with me, and it had been a great strain to put on a happy face and to conceal from her (on Mary Louise's directive) any suggestion of what was going on.

It was only after I arranged to meet at Dr. L.'s office in the morning that Mary Louise told me what he'd said to her.

"I wonder why he told me that?" she said. "Why is he so insistent in trying to deprive me of all hope?"

I was enraged. I was convinced without any doubt that the doctor had *never* given anyone the substance. And if he believed his AMA propaganda and thought it worthless, why not convey the thought to me rather than to the patient? The more I thought about it, the angrier I became.

I met with him the next morning at 8:30. It was a Sunday morning. I had brought along a great deal of the medical literature on the subject.

"All I want you to do is to show me how to inject the stuff," I said. "And I want you to stop lying. You told Mary Louise you had tried Krebiozen with other patients, and you know you've never used it before in your life!"

He tried to insist that he had used it.

"Stop the horseshit. You've never used it before in your life!"

As he pretended to study the literature, he kept insisting. Finally he said: "I had it given—"

"You didn't give it and you didn't have it given," I said flatly.

A short time later, he said: "You listen to me. I had it given by Dr. Durovic to six or seven patients at Trafalgar Hospital."

I pointed an angry finger at him: "Now you listen to me," I said. "Dr. Durovic never practiced in New York in his entire life—and therefore never set foot in Trafalgar Hospital!"

He made another feeble attempt to defend his lie.

"What I don't understand is how you could be such a shit as to tell your lies to my wife behind my back," I said. "Now, let me ask you something. You wouldn't give any substance to a patient without reading the literature first, would you?"

Even as he answered, "Of course not. That's why I'm reading this," his face fell, for he realized he'd fallen into a trap.

"Exactly," I said. "You're reading the literature because you haven't read it before. And you certainly wouldn't have injected the substance in anyone without reading it."

Although the literature pointed out that the substance was nontoxic and that 4,000 physicians and surgeons had used it, the doctor said he would not give it "outside of a hospital."

"You're doing a terrible thing," I told him. "You are her only doctor and you're abandoning her. Be certain that either I'll find someone to inject this or I'll do it myself—"

"I'm sure you will," he said. "If I can be helpful after that—"

The little worm was afraid that he had lost all future fees. And indeed he had.

It was difficult breaking the news to Mary Louise. I remembered the woman quack she'd gone to. We made arrangements to go to her office—a distance of some forty miles. Dr. Quack made an injection, gave me an unlimited prescription for needles, and showed me carefully how to administer injections myself.

For five days, we tried the substance. Mary Louise was running a fever (oral) of 105 and was in considerable pain. Nevertheless, the injections seemed to coincide with an immediate return of her appetite, which she had almost totally lost.

No one, even its staunchest advocates, has ever claimed that "Carcalon" helps more than 30% of those to whom it is given. Perhaps it needed more of a chance—but time was beginning to run out. . . .

I investigated what had seemed like the worth-while responses to my ad. Hope fell apart.

One letter continued to bother me. It was from a prominent theatrical attorney. She wrote: "Firstly, I want it clearly understood that the offer of $25,000 is more of a deterrent than a lure in-sofar as the research in which I am so deeply interested is concerned. . . . The treatment is given by a dedicated physician licensed to practice in New York who refuses fees or emoluments in any form for his services. . . ."

I contacted her. She was delighted to learn who had placed the ad in the *Times*, for it seems that I was one of her "heroes"—I had written about her doctor in *The Independent* some fourteen years before!

I met with the doctor. He insisted on two con-ditions. He would accept no money for medication or service . . . and I must promise not to give any publicity to the fact that he was treating her. Thus, what follows regarding him is limited by my pledge to him.

I cannot even discuss his theory or his approach. He is a warm, sensitive man with a fantastic grasp of medicine. He is undoubtedly something of a genius.

I spoke to two physicians whose lives he had saved.

He visited our apartment in Brooklyn. He made some perceptive observations but few promises. On the contrary, when I drove him home he explained how hopeless the condition was in a "young" person. If Mary Louise had been thirty years older, it would take a year for growth to take place that would now take a couple of weeks to a month.

Nevertheless, after some tests, he became more encouraging. He had told Mary Louise he saved "about fifty percent" of cases with liver involvement. She was quite hopeful.

We began with his medication and her pain began to disappear. Her appetite increased considerably. She was able to sleep again. Her fever dropped to 101 and he insisted that it would drop to below 100. It did.

He was to visit her two weeks later. Each morning precisely at 9:15 we telephoned him and reported on various tests, disorders, changes. As the two weeks flew by, she looked forward eagerly to his next visit. She was troubled by the fact that nobody could tell her whether the tumor was still growing.

She came to the verge of tears once and she cried once.

We had been discussing the future and somehow the conversation turned morbidly on the fact that if she died of this thing, the tragedy would be that she wouldn't be around to see the things that I might still accomplish or to see Rory John grow into manhood.

"You'd better stop," she said, "or I'm going to cry."

The occasion on which she cried was during the American Booksellers Convention in Washington. I had been the first publisher ever to take his family to the conventions and we hadn't missed one in eight years. Now she couldn't be there.

Sandra Lee came in from Wisconsin. She spent the day with her mother, and her mother told her.

Rory John had already been told.

I flew to Washington for a few hours to break the news to her sister, Eileen.

Nobody could quite believe it.

Early in May I had sold a small percentage of

our book-publishing business for half a million dollars. On the day that I brought the check home to show it to her she expressed concern that I had made the sale to pay for her Jamaica house or to pay her medical bills and had compromised my independence. I assured her that that wasn't remotely so and that I still retained a considerable majority of the stock, and total control of my business and all publishing decisions.

We then decided to give some stock to each of our employees who had been with us for more than two years. She co-signed the gift letters with me.

I racked my brain to figure out how our "fresh" money could provide her with comfort.

The answer came. She had been depressed because it was obvious that we were no longer going to make our July 1 journey to Jamaica.

Why not? If she could lie in a bed in Brooklyn, why couldn't she lie in a bed in Jamaica?

I set the machinery in motion. Transportation to the airport. A stretcher on the plane. An ambulance from Montego Bay to Bolt House in Port Maria.

There were all sorts of technical problems. BOAC had booked the flight but we were taking an Air Jamaica plane.

Meanwhile, a good friend who is, I believe, a good doctor, visited us.

"She doesn't have a chance," he said. "I doubt if she will live three weeks. My advice is to forget Jamaica and get her into a hospital."

"She hates hospitals," I said.

"I don't care. Get her into one and get round-the-clock nurses. Get her under narcotics so she doesn't know what is happening. She shouldn't have to endure pain."

But her pain seemed to be diminishing.

Another doctor, Robert Kamen, who'd married one of my childhood friends, was called in for a consultation.

"You say a doctor told you 'three weeks'? She may not even have that long. The tumor is growing rapidly. I don't know why she has so little pain but I'm afraid it will return and then some. I'll prescribe a euphoric. I suggest you give it to her at once."

According to the theory of the doctor who was treating her, narcotics could not be used because they not only dulled pain but also deadened the ability of the body to resist.

There was another factor. She was alive only so long as she was conscious. When she went to narcotics, she would become a vegetable. It was living death.

The doctors didn't see it that way. But, then, they weren't in love with her.

Her doctor was to see her again in three days. It would be his second visit: they had met but once.

One morning, when we made our regular 9:15 a.m. phone call, there was no answer.

"He's sick," Mary Louise said.

"Don't be silly, honey," I assured her. "Just because he doesn't answer the phone doesn't mean he's sick. It could be any of a number of things."

"He's sick," she said.

His nurse called. He was at home with a gall bladder attack. He was all right and would be in touch.

"It's a heart attack," Mary Louise said.

It was a heart attack.

That evening he got to a phone (against his own physician's instructions) and spoke to her. He didn't miss a day. Two days later, they took him to the hospital. He would phone her daily. But he obviously wasn't going to be able to examine her personally again for some time. She was depressed about this.

She never saw him again.

He was against our going to Jamaica. I pointed out that we would phone him each morning just as we had been doing. There would be no difference except that she would have pleasanter surroundings, cleaner air, and a friendlier atmosphere.

We got her to the airport. Four of the fellows who work with us—three of them Puerto Ricans—carried her on the stretcher, ever so gently.

Air Jamaica had forgotten to provide a stretcher.

We overcame this crisis by tying our own stretcher to the seats. We had booked first class. This meant that we would pay double fare for her and she would occupy two first-class seats. But Air Jamaica said this was their first stretcher case and they would only carry her at the back of the plane.

The back of the plane was empty. It became necessary to turn down sixteen seats to accommodate the stretcher.

The ambulance waiting at Montego Bay was a farce. It was twenty years old. Or seemed like it. There was no ventilation. There was carburetor trouble. On the way it had a flat tire.

While Mary Louise lay in the hot ambulance, I tried to muster our things through Jamaica customs. This is the one customs service in the world which treats visiting Americans as potential thieves, smugglers, and revolutionaries. It took one-half hour to clear.

Port Maria is 85 miles from Montego Bay. Halfway there our car and the ambulance stopped for gas.

"By the way, how much will this be?" I asked the ambulance owner-driver.

"Well, I think a dollar a mile would be fair."

"It's eighty-five miles. Eighty-five dollars."

"No," he said. "I think it's nearer ninety-five miles. And you've got to include the trip from Kingston and back again. That makes about two hundred and fifty miles."

"Are you trying to say that you want $250 for this two-and-one-half-hour ride?"

That's what he was trying to say. I later learned that the charge should have been $70. I ended up paying him $140—happy that we had arrived at Bolt House at last.

I will always be grateful to Blanche Blackwell for her Bolt House.

Almost from the day we arrived, Mary Louise began to brighten up.

The picture window in the beautiful bedroom gave her a sweeping view of the spectacular terrain. The pool was outside her window and the children and visiting friends could wave to her and blow kisses to her.

I talked to the staff. I told them candidly what the problems were. I told them that, although this was the first time Bolt had ever been rented, I was sure they knew that staff usually hoped for tips from the guests when they departed and wondered all month if they would get them and how large they would be. I said that I was a generous tipper but that I wouldn't keep them in suspense. I was going to pay them each week the same amount of money that Bolt was paying them. They would receive double their salaries.

The first weeks . . . friends came and went. They would wave to her in our air-conditioned bedroom from the picture window facing the pool. Cook was the greatest and Mary Louise ate ravenously. In the beginning she made an attempt to sit at the dining room table with us for one course, at least.

The house was a terrible problem: our house, that is. There was no water—nor any provision for a supply. The phone company said they couldn't give us a phone for now—there were no facilities. The road was virtually impassable. There was no electric power and the company was talking about engineering a plan and it would cost me about $4,500 to bring power to our house. The things we had bought in Denmark had arrived and were on the dock but we learned that it is against regulations to import furniture into Jamaica—new furniture, that is. An order of household things from Sears was similarly being held up.

Let me elaborate on two of perhaps sixteen problems. Electricity. I made the mountainous drive to Kingston to the Public Service Company. It takes two hours each way. In Kingston, I was told that I was at the wrong place. "You should go to St. Ann's Bay," they said. (I noticed that of the hundreds of typewriters in the place, not one was electric. The Public Service Company knows its own limitations better than anyone.) I went to St. Ann's Bay. "Oh, no," I was told. "You should have gone to Kingston."

"But I've been to Kingston and they told me to come here."

"Well . . . we can't help you."

Water: Three applications had been "lost" over an eight-month period. The fourth was on file. No action had been taken. My solicitor (lawyer) had accomplished nothing. A meeting was arranged with Parish Council officials and a member of parliament. The M.P. expressed great surprise that people had been so unconcerned. He recognized the water need as an emergency situation. He would get a special appropriation from Kingston. He did. But by the time it became official, four weeks passed. By the time work began, another two weeks passed. We were given a small daily supply of water by truck.

I insisted that the water line go not just up to my property but all the way up the road to Grant's Town. I wanted the poor people in the area to benefit by our coming to Jamaica. At last there was a compromise. A four-inch pipe would go to our property and three-inch pipe after that to Grant's

Town. My neighbors came to thank me. Some of them had been promised water for nine years. . . .

Want a couple of others? Each morning I had to reach Mary Louise's physician in New York. One out of six mornings, the phone was completely out of service for the day. Other mornings, it would take more than 100 rings (yes, I counted them) to get an overseas operator.

Once when I complained, an operator told me: "We are only six and we must handle the entire country. We are not out having tea as people suggest."

To get an operator or to get to another town, you dialed a code. All codes began with "0". Thus, the overseas operator code was "000" and the trunk operator "008". (It was in Oracabessa that Ian Fleming picked up his James Bond agent number, "007", for that was the Oracabessa exchange code.) So you dialed the first "0" and you got a busy signal. And no matter what the emergency—if you didn't get past the first "0" you didn't reach *anybody*.

The Ministry of Trade and Industry is a whole comic farce in itself. Its job is to "protect Jamaican industry" by restricting imports on things that are manufactured in Jamaica.

Now, with lower labor costs . . . no shipping

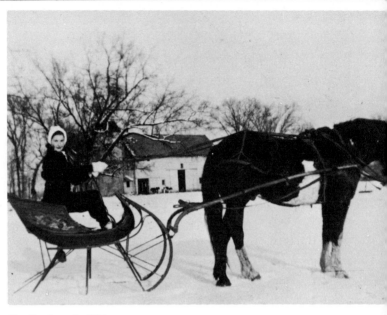

On the farm in Ohio

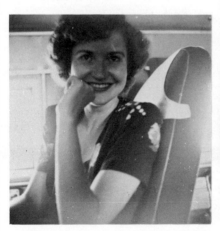

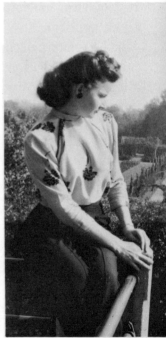

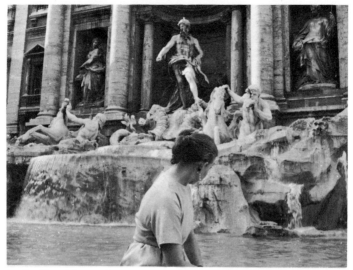

At the Trevi Fountain

Mary Louise and Sandy

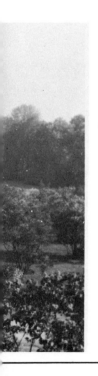

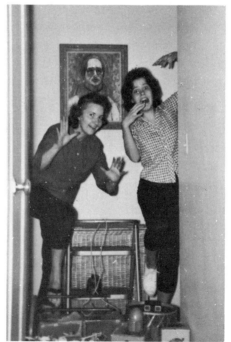

costs . . . one would think that, on a purely competitive basis, Jamaican industry would thrive. Nobody is taking that chance.

Let a company announce that they are going to build a plant to process tomato juice and the next day no tomato juice is allowed into the island! Mind you, the plant doesn't exist yet: not a brick has been laid. This actually happened and is typical.

Item upon item can't be bought in Jamaica. The things aren't being made there. But it is against the law to import them.

Duty on allowable imports staggers the purse. It runs to 71½% on American automobiles and 49% on British-made cars. Almost every new product is heavily taxed. Thus, when a friend brought a $14 hair dryer to Jamaica for Mary Louise, the customs inspector spotted it in her luggage, saw that it was new, and taxed her $6.

I was told we couldn't bring the Danish furniture into Jamaica.

My solicitor called one evening. "You must go to Kingston tomorrow morning early. The customs broker may be able to solve the problems."

I hated to leave Mary Louise for another full day, although there were others on hand to look after her. Nevertheless, I left the house at 6 a.m. and arrived at Kingston at 8. The office didn't open until 9. I went there at 9:15. The man I had come to see had gone out "for a short while." He didn't return until 1 p.m.

Then began a comic chase. We had to go to four government offices to apply for permission to import things. One man for towels. Another for glasses. The Sears order said "3 diapers" (actually, there were three dozen) and this required a conference to see if diapers could be imported at all. (We use them for dust rags.) Finally we were told we could import the "3 diapers" but would have to apply for trade board approval.

Had enough? I did. Up to my eyelashes. I was so disgusted with things that I seriously considered destroying what had been built so far on our property and abandoning the place.

Mary Louise, depressed by what it was doing to me, thought about it for a day. Then she suggested that we allow the place to be finished and simply put it on the market for sale.

(The outcome of the import thing? We were fined $60 for not having applied for permission *before* buying the furniture. Then we were taxed customs duty of about $2,400 on merchandise for which we had paid no more than $3,500.)

I had no leverage. In the States there are people to consult with. There are friends to call. Officials to pressure. Something. The frustrations mounted and there was nothing to do.

A private intelligence agent was hired by a major hotel to "evaluate" the situation as regards the black militant movement, revolutionary movements, etc., on the island. The hotel owners wanted to know, before putting more money into their property.

The agent quickly infiltrated. He reported a couple of weeks later that the militants and revolutionaries would seem to pose no threat. They were disorganized and without much of a plan. Except for one thing: the government was even more disorganized! (The hotel owners decided to make no further investment.)

The political party in power is now fragmented into three groups and the result is that nobody dares to make a decision because to do nothing seems safer than to do something and be open to criticism for it.

Animated discussion often takes place in Port Maria on whether the phone service is worse than the electric company or vice versa. The phone billing system is so bad that the town was being charged a few hundred pounds too much and refused to pay unless the charges were itemized. Instead, the phone company cut off service so that you could call the Fire Department but they couldn't make any outgoing calls.

The Hardware Merchants' Association published

a full-page ad in the Jamaica paper (*The Daily Gleaner*) apologizing for the fact that hardware stores were no longer able to supply locks, hinges, latches, etc. It seems that one company had gone into the hardware-manufacturing business and the government had immediately banned all imports. The ad reminded readers that ". . . no one factory in any part of the world could hope to produce a full range of *all* the types, designs, variations and finishes of *all* these items. In hinges alone there would be perhaps about 300 sizes, shapes, types and finishes. . . ."

For four weeks, Mary Louise seemed to be holding her own beautifully. Pain seemed to be under control and, according to the local surgeon whom I had hired to examine her, she showed none of the symptoms that she should have shown with her condition. He was startled and amazed.

I, on the other hand, was startled and amazed at what the human body could endure. Mary Louise had to take three kinds of medication, every hour of the day and night. I found myself getting a half hour's sleep and then gingerly leaping out of the bed to count the drops, filling capsules, pouring water.

At the end of a week I was groggy. I felt a desperate need for uninterrupted sleep. For, in addition to being a kind of on-the-spot nurse, I was also trying to direct the household, keep guests entertained, and push our own house toward completion.

There are few nurses available on the island. I managed to obtain one from 9 p.m. to 6 a.m. I asked Mary Louise's sister to join me, and the two of us shared the daily nursing chores.

At this point, no one faltered in the belief that somehow she was going to pull through. The tumor didn't seem to be growing. Her appetite was good. There was no sign of jaundice.

When the pain began again, she bore it stoically.

Each morning we would call New York and each morning the doctor reassured her and had something for her to do: increase the drops of this or discontinue that. Eat this or don't eat that.

The pain became rougher. Soon, someone was always massaging her feet and her legs.

"That seems to help," she would say.

We would powder her down or give her an alcohol rub. Always slowly and gently.

She remarked once: "Do you know, I don't think I could stand the pain without all of this special attention."

Another time: "For the first time in my life I have no desire to return to our Brooklyn apartment. In fact, if I knew I had only a month to live, I'd want to live it here."

We rented Bolt House for August. The plan now was to stay through the summer and, on August 28, to return to New York and put her in a hospital.

Avant Keels came to Jamaica. He is black and one of my two oldest friends. It was his $400 added to our $1,000 that launched *The Independent* in November, 1951. She held his hand. "Friendship is a very wonderful thing," she said.

Lori and Cheri Leffert came separately. They gave the place new cheer. They are both extraordinary young ladies. They would tell Mary Louise how beautiful she looked. They would comb her hair and hold her hand.

Soon, someone was holding her hand almost all the time.

Carlos Gonzalez and his girl friend departed. Paul and Barbara Schumer came and went. Avant. Terry Garrity.

Her sister, Eileen, went back to Florida, only to return in a few days. While home, she told their father for the first time of Mary Louise's illness. He is eighty. A short time later, he called Eileen.

"I've been thinking," he said. "I'm an old man and I don't really need my liver. . . ."

Eileen explained that that wasn't the solution. We told Mary Louise and she smiled.

Our daughter Sandra Lee arrived. Sandy had

not realized how serious the illness had become. Mary Louise felt that nothing was to be gained by depressing those she loved.

Bill Gaines, that sweetheart of a fellow, flew to Jamaica for just two days so he could say hello to her and cheer her up. Then he was off to take his *Mad* staff on a ten-day tour of Africa.

She hated and dreaded hospitals. At the Ocho Rios airport Bill turned to me: "I would think twice before I would take her back to New York. Particularly unless you're sure they can do something for her there that you can't do for her here."

Her backbone had begun to protrude. Her arms had become concentration-camp thin. Only her beautiful face was full and untouched.

Lying in bed was so uncomfortable for her that she would ask to be sat up again and again. Eileen once counted twenty-five times in thirty minutes. We would, each time, fix pillows under her knees, at her feet, under her head. And then take them all out again and pull her up. We tried everything.

"Can you straighten me out?" she would say. "Could you raise me just an inch?"

There were never demands. It was always a gentle request.

To Rory John, to whom she had always said: "I love you," she now began to say, "I love you *so much*."

One day I came into the room and Eileen was crying. Mary Louise had been talking with her and had said: "I guess I'm not saying what I want to say. I guess all I want to say is that I love you."

When I walked in, Mary Louise was patting Eileen's hand and she said to me, "Eileen is feeling bad."

In July she had done considerable reading. Books were too heavy for her to hold so I would tear the pages out and she would read a few pages at a time. She particularly enjoyed *The Kingdom and the Power* (about the *New York Times*), found Pearl Buck's new novel interesting, and was disappointed in a novel called *The Board Room*. She started to read *Exodus* and would tell Rory John some of the story. She managed it down to the last dozen pages, when the pain made it too difficult to concentrate on reading.

She never finished the book.

The nurse couldn't make it every night and we managed to obtain a substitute. The local doctor was persuaded to make a daily visit. The doctor in New York expressed alarm at her new symptoms and urged me to return her to New York. It wasn't that easy: the planes were booked to capacity for weeks in advance. August 28 was our day and we would have to hold to it.

When I talked with her I talked about "when you get well again, we'll do thus and so. . . ."

One night she told her nurse (I didn't learn this until afterward) : "I'm trying to live a year for my husband but I don't think I'm going to make it."

The substitute nurse was a sweet young girl named Veronica Braham who even as a child had dressed as a nurse and nursed her dolls. She was excellent. Mary Louise liked her, so I persuaded her to join us on the trip back to New York and to work at the hospital on one shift a day.

Veronica had been to India. She talked with Mary Louise about Yoga. They talked about the Yoga approach to illness.

"Peace is the first step in Yoga," Veronica said.

Mary Louise smiled. "I'll try that."

The local doctor, son of the local surgeon who had first examined her in Jamaica, was Dr. Philip Harry. He had been practicing medicine for two years and was competent and conscientious. After conferring with the doctor in New York, he tapped her abdomen and later her lung. He was convinced the cancer had reached her lung. But taking out a large amount of fluid gave her relief and she could breathe again without gasping.

I had done my homework as a journalist. I knew that the doctor in New York controlled not "half" of his cancer patients but perhaps one in two hundred. He did, however, enable them to live longer. And—they seemed able to live without narcotics and so be living human beings instead of half-conscious vegetables.

I knew too (but never told Mary Louise) that the doctor in New York hadn't been able to save his own wife when she had cancer four years before. He had followed the same discipline: no narcotics. He felt that, once narcotics are begun, there is no hope at all. Without them, there is always hope of some peculiar remission. He'd had the experience and the living patients to prove it.

She could no longer leave the bed. I hired a five-piece Jamaican orchestra to play on our terrace and we carried her into the living room on a stretcher. At other times we carried her out to watch the glorious evening as the full moon shimmered on the tropical sea.

By mid-August she began to fade. The changes were subtle and then not so subtle. She began to eat less. She suffered more. A slight yellow began to show in the whites of her eyes.

"I would have given up weeks ago," her sister said.

"I don't understand how she can bear the pain without narcotics," Dr. Harry remarked. "She seems to be living on pure will."

Six days to go until departure time. . . .
That day her skin had indicated that her liver was no longer able to produce vitamin "K" and the doctor gave her an injection of it.

She hadn't slept for two days and asked the doctor if he had anything that would permit her to sleep. He gave her a vitamin and enzyme combination. I dropped into his office in Port Maria for the pills and then made the 40-mile round trip to Ocho Rios to search the town for some disposable diapers. I found them.

On Friday evening, she had Eileen phone to Dr. Harry to ask if there wasn't anything he could do to help her leg, which was aching so terribly throughout. This in itself was most unusual. She was so self-controlled that in the past she would list her pains and ailments and report them during the doctor's regular visit.

She was due to be taken to the new house in the morning. It was now finished and Eileen and Rory and Sandy had worked hard and long to arrange the furniture.

At 9 p.m. the nurse arrived and I went to the room I shared with Rory to get some sleep. The

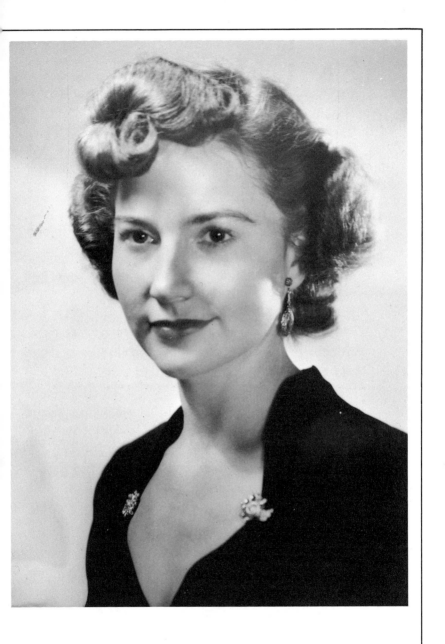

nurse woke me at 10:30. Mary Louise wanted to be moved.

I carried her to one of the other beds. Then back to the hospital bed again.

Now she looked at me, and in a language that only a couple who have loved each other for twenty-three years could understand, said, "Can you help me?" Her voice was plaintive, almost apologetic.

"I'm going to give you one of those narcotic tablets we got from Dr. Kamen. Just one."

"Will it help me?"

"It will help you to sleep and you haven't slept for three days. We're not going to do it as a regular thing but this time it's all right."

"If you say so," she said.

I gave her a tablet, but still she couldn't sleep. After half an hour she said, "Could I have just another half pill?"

"I'll give you another whole one," I said. I did.

She slept for a few hours.

I was awakened again at 3:30 a.m. She wanted to be moved to the other bed. The pills had indeed killed the pain.

As she came out of sleep, she said, "Are we having another adventure?"

"Yes, sweetie," I said, "and you just relax."

At another time she said: "What marshmallow?"

"Try to get some more sleep, sweetie," I said. "Close your eyes and I'll rest my chin on your bed and close my eyes and we'll both sleep."

"Will that be good for me?" she asked.

"Yes," I assured her.

I lay my head on the side of the bed and closed my eyes.

"You're cheating!" she said suddenly with a cute smile on her face. "You closed your eyes before I closed mine."

"Okay," I said, "you close yours first."

"I think it would be better if you don't close yours," she explained. "I feel a sense of panic about orienting myself again and I'd like you to watch me."

When Eileen came into the room in the morning, she heard Mary Louise say to me: "Does she know we cheated?"

The narcotic hadn't completely worn off. She spoke about looking forward to the ambulance ride and, when the ambulance I had hired arrived to take her to the new house, her eyes were half closed.

It was the morning of August 23. *Five days to go until our return to New York.*

When the ambulance reached the Stuart place, I had two of the strongest men on the island standing by to carry the stretcher through the house. We took her up the stairs to the master bedroom. We showed her the living room.

"It's beautiful," she said to Eileen and the kids. "You've done a beautiful job."

Then she wanted to be taken back to Bolt. Without seeing the kitchen or the playroom or the guest house.

Returning to Bolt I reminded her that she had said she looked forward to the ambulance ride.

"Yes," she said, "because it helps me to sleep."

I reminded her too that she hadn't seen the kitchen, which was now perfect.

She smiled and squeezed my hand. "But I know everything that's in it," she said.

Her eyes were much more yellowed. She had stopped eating solid food and was living on Sustagen.

Later that morning her sister Eileen sat beside her while her daughter Sandra and I drove to Ocho Rios to buy more Chux.

Eileen reports that at one point she asked: "Eileen, what are we trying to accomplish? Just what is our objective?"

"We're waiting for Lyle to get back from Ocho Rios and for you to get some sleep so you can get well."

"If I'm to wait until Lyle gets back from Ocho Rios and to go to sleep and get better, then why don't you stop poking me?"

Eileen hadn't touched her. Mary Louise had been feeling her own legs with her hands. The narcotic obviously hadn't worn off.

There had been blood in her stool. When I reported this to her New York physician, he took her off all medication except a preparation to control bleeding.

That afternoon and early evening she didn't want me to leave her side. When Sandy came in to relieve me, Mary Louise said, "Stay with me a few minutes more."

"But, honey, Sandy is a good nurse."

"Sandy is a great nurse," she replied, "but you stay with me a little while longer."

I sat next to her bed, holding her hand. From time to time she would say, "Would you pick me up, please?" I'd sit her up. Almost at once, she would want to lie down again.

Dinnertime. I made ready to place the large bell at her fingertips. "I have to go to supper now, honey."

"Could you stay with me now and eat later?" she asked plaintively.

This was unlike her. But I was too exhausted, too sleep-starved to recognize that something was happening. She continued to shift positions and I continued to do the many things I'd learned to do to try to make her more comfortable.

The effects of the narcotic had just about worn off completely. Earlier in the day she had remarked to Eileen: "I think I'm going to find out where I'm at, later today."

"How am I going to get myself feeling better?" she asked, just before the night nurse arrived.

I went to sleep in the master bed in her room with the nurse sitting by watching her. It was 9 p.m.

At 10:30 I was awakened. She wanted to be moved to another bed. Usually I lifted her and carried her, but now she wanted to walk herself. The nurse and I each held one side and walk-carried her to the bed. There was the usual ritual of fixing pillows and blankets, and then she said she wanted to be moved to the master bed. This time again she insisted on trying to walk with our support. I got into bed with her, for it was the bed in which I'd been sleeping.

After many changes, I reminded her that we'd been moving the pillows around "sixteen times."

"Could you try once more?" she asked.

Throughout her illness, it had been necessary for her to lie on her back. Now, suddenly, she turned on her side—something she hadn't done in months.

"Perhaps it would help if you'd cuddle me," she said.

I put my arms around her and hugged her. We kissed. After a moment she announced that she wanted to be returned to the hospital bed at the window. Again she insisted on walking with the nurse and me supporting her.

I lay my chin on the side of her bed. "Sweetie, tomorrow your father and Edna and your Aunt May [her favorite aunt] are coming. I've got to get some sleep or I won't be any good to you or to them. I'll go to Rory's room and I'll be back in just a few hours."

We kissed again. It was about 11:30.

At 12:30, she called to the nurse, "Would you wipe me, please?"

She had begun to hemorrhage from the rectum.

"I'll go call Mr. Stuart," the nurse said, when she saw what was happening.

"No, don't bother him. Let him sleep," she said.

The nurse rapped at my door. I raced after her back to the room. The nurse summoned the local doctor. I raced outside to phone her physician in New York. It took an eternity to reach an overseas operator.

The physician directed an immediate injection and also two tablespoons of medicine orally. She dutifully swallowed the medicine.

She wanted to sit up and the nurse seemed to want her to lie still.

"You have to believe me," Mary Louise said, "I must sit up."

We sat her up. I wakened Eileen and Sandy.

By the time Dr. Harry hurried into the bedroom, she was sitting in a pool of blood and there was a gurgling sound in her throat.

"She's dying," the nurse said.

Mary Louise looked at me, a frightened little-girl expression on her face. "What did she say?" she asked.

"Nothing, honey!" I said. I was hugging her to me and kissing her cheek. "I love you! I love you! Don't leave me!"

It was the last thing she heard. The gurgling grew louder and she hemorrhaged from the mouth. She didn't recognize Dr. Harry as he took over. He worked hard but somehow everyone in the room knew she was dead.

It was 1 a.m. Sunday, August 24.

She was my wife and my sweetheart. She was a most wonderful wife. As everyone knew who knew us, I adored her.

A few weeks before, I had told her that I had really come to know my motivation. I was *so* proud of her—so proud of the way she looked and the way she talked and the way she thought and the things she did—so proud. . . .

And I wanted so much to make her proud of me.

That had been my motivation from the time we met in Columbus, Ohio, nearly a quarter of a century before.

She was the only woman I have ever truly loved. She was not just my angel—she was everybody's angel. Words like "beautiful," "fascinating," "brilliant," "radiant," "warm," "perceptive," "gentle," "courageous"—all these and many more couldn't half begin to paint her picture.

She was my wife and the mother of my children. Quite apart from any of this, *she was the most remarkable person I have ever known.*

Some weeks before, while she was enduring a particularly severe bout with pain, I told her what my friend and former high school teacher Philip Roddman had said about her. "She is," he'd said, "the only civilized woman I've ever met."

Overcoming her agony for a moment, she managed a bright smile. "Philip is a doll!" she said.

She loved her children. She had tried to pass on to them the rational, sensible attitudes toward things that she shared with me.

(A few nights before, the nurse had begun to tell her that she should put her faith in god. "Oh, no!" she laughed. "I used to believe that when I was a very little girl but I stopped believing that when I grew up and I'm too old to begin believing now!")

Sandra Lee had been with us at the moment of her death. But Rory John was still asleep. How could I tell *him,* our thirteen-year-old who adored her and whom she adored? Do I wake him now and tell him through my tears or do I allow him his needed sleep and tell him in the morning?

I needed advice. I needed Mary Louise. For the first time in twenty-three years she wasn't there— and I didn't know what to do.

Her sister, Eileen, urged that I wake him right away.

I walked into his room. I wasn't sure I was doing the right thing. For twenty-three years, when I needed advice, she had told me the right thing to do.

The doctor called a crematory in Kingston. They told him they'd be at Bolt House in two hours.

I sat in the room with her. A few rooms away, I could hear Rory John howling uncontrollably, but his sister and his aunt were with him and Dr. Harry was getting ready to give him the sedative he'd asked for.

We had often discussed the fact that we cry at the death of someone because of our own loss.

A few weeks before, she had said: "People make too much of death. When I die, perhaps you should throw a party."

Rory and Sandy have their lives ahead of them. They are well fortified. She gave meaning to the word "character" and some of it has obviously rubbed off on them.

I would "recover" . . . everyone does, don't they? I would act out the charade that is business and the charade that is social life.

The men who had given me all that money for a small chunk of my business had been patient and understanding. And they had made it possible for Mary Louise to have every comfort money could buy. I would make the business thrive for them.

But these are obligations. There are no more motivations. She is dead and I am on my way to death and the world is a dead place for me.

Oh my love, my love—how you suffered—and I so helpless—so unable to help. . . .

Last spring we had planned to take the children to Ohio by car. I hadn't been back to Columbus since 1946 and we would show them where she was born and where she grew up and the farm outside of Milford Center. For the journey I had rented a large automobile because the small ones we drive wouldn't be pleasant on long highway driving.

The car is still in the garage. It has barely been used.

When I was courting her in Columbus, there was

a popular song lyric based on some lines from Shakespeare which ended:

"You and I will journey on,
  we are but the stuff that dreams are built upon
Others in our place will face the skies again
  then you and I forever and forever will rise
    again
For though our little dream is ended in a sleep
Don't weep, the stars remain."

A few weeks before, suffering excruciating pain, she had said, "If only I could cry. It would be a release if only I could cry."

"Cry, sweetie," I had said. "Don't be ashamed to cry."

"I can't," she said. "Ever since childhood I've trained myself not to cry and now I can't."

The crematory acts in typical Jamaican style. After 3½ hours, the nurse telephones Kingston.

"You said you would be here in two hours," she says.

They have no record of the original call. They will send someone now.

The sun is rising when they come to take the body.

Her father, stepmother, and aunt arrived a few hours later.

When her mother became ill, we took the first flight to Florida. When we arrived, she had died.

Now her father arrives and his daughter is dead.

The telephone isn't working. I can't get past the first "0" to notify New York. It isn't until the next morning that I am able to call, and that, only by driving to Port Maria and using the public phone booth in the street.

Bob Salomon answers my private line. "Hey! Guess what!" he says. "We have *two* books on the best-seller list next week! *Captive City* and *Naked Came the Stranger* are both on the list!"

"Good," I say, thinking that Mary Louise would be pleased about that. "Bob, let me speak to Carole."

I try to contain myself as I say to my secretary and publicity director Carole Livingston, "Carole, take this list of names." I begin to reel them off.

My mind flashes back to the week before when, during excruciating pain, Mary Louise had said, "Oh, dear, whatever will I do?"

Now, as I come to the end of the long list, I say, "Tell these people that Mary Louise died in my arms yesterday morning." And my voice breaks and I hear myself sobbing, "Oh Carole, Carole. Whatever will I do? Whatever will I do?"

I hang up and walk from the booth, crying openly, unashamedly. The local blacks on the main street stare at the weeping white man. They know. Everybody knows everything that happens here in Port Maria.

Monday passes. In the evening, I speak to Dr. Harry. He asks if I have registered the death with the police. Until I do that, they can't cremate her.

Horrified, I phone the crematory. No, they haven't cremated her. I didn't register the death yet, did I?

I assure them I'll do it the first thing Tuesday morning but they say they are "fully booked" for Tuesday and couldn't burn her till Wednesday. Only after intense pressure from me do they agree to "try to fit her in."

I speak to them on Tuesday morning. Later they call to tell me the cremation is half-done. It takes three hours altogether. I can send for the ashes now.

I drive to the Playboy to find Clyde Satterthwaite. He was the taxi driver who drove her to Kingston when she was with Faye Fingesten and who drove us to Kingston when we were in Jamaica together in May. He was her favorite and I know that he is the one I have to send for her ashes.

Eileen receives the package. We do not mention specifics to the children or to her father. They have enough to be depressed about.

Eileen places the package next to my typewriter in what I have begun to call "her room."

I sleep there, alone in the house. The others are sleeping in the guest house at the Stuart place.

"I can still smell her blood in the room," I tell Eileen.

"Sandy and I thought we did too but then we thought it must be our imagination," Eileen says.

From Bolt House to "the Stuart place" it is a mile and a quarter by foot.

At 3 a.m. I awaken and dress. There is no car available to me and I must walk. I carry the package of ashes close to me and walk slowly through the night.

A man, walking beside his bicycle, passes me going the other way. "Good morning, boss," he says. "Taking your early morning walk?"

"Good morning," I say.

I pass Noel Coward's Blue Harbor—the house on the sea that he uses for guests. At last I reach Parochial Road #194 and turn to the right to climb its rocky, winding trail.

It isn't five o'clock yet, but three men are already digging into the earth to make way for the water pipe that will carry the water supply to the community. They get paid by the chain and are anxious to dig as much as they can before the hot sun comes up.

"Good morning, Mr. Stuart," one of them says.
"Good morning."

Her words echo in my mind. "People make too much of death. When I die, perhaps you should throw a party."

I walk through the rooms of the new house—*her* house—carrying the package. To her powder room with its fabulous light fixture and the dressing table with the five-foot-wide mirror and the line of theatrical-like light bulbs on each side. To the terrace that looks out over one of the most breathtaking panoramic views in the world. The central air conditioner is going now—just as if someone lived here. I walk from the bedroom to the study she had built for me. There is a standup desk because she thought it would be healthful for me. And there is the handsome custom-crafted mahoe desk—a double desk with an Eames chair on each side. It was here that we would have worked together, facing each other.

The shadows are lifting and daylight is coming, all too fast. I open the package and begin sprinkling the ashes. In the planters that will hold the lovely ferns and flowers. And then, all about the grounds that surrounded her beautiful house.

On the wall of the powder room at Bolt House hangs a copy of a poem published by Noel Coward in a limited edition for his friends. He wrote it in 1966.

Nothing Is Lost*

Deep in our sub-conscious, we are told
Lie all our memories, lie all the notes
Of all the music we have ever heard
And all the phrases those we loved have spoken,
Sorrows and losses time has since consoled,
Family jokes, out-moded anecdotes
Each sentimental souvenir and token
Everything seen, experienced, each word
Addressed to us in infancy, before . . .
Before we could even know or understand
The implications of our wonderland.
There they all are, the legendary lies
The birthday treats, the sights, the sounds, the tears
Forgotten debris of forgotten years
Waiting to be recalled, waiting to rise
Before our world dissolves before our eyes
Waiting for some small intimate reminder,
A word, a tune, a known familiar scent
An echo from the past when, innocent
We looked upon the present with delight
And doubted not the future would be kinder
And never knew the loneliness of night.

And now I was to know the loneliness of night.

Oh my darling, my precious darling! You lit up my whole world. You took me by the hand and led

* © 1966 Noel Coward.

me out of the darkness and now the lights have gone out and there's nothing ahead . . . nothing.

The *Times* is kind enough to publish her obituary on the page facing the book page. And on the same page is our announcement that the office will be closed on the morrow in her memory . . . "Lyle Stuart Inc. which she co-founded and inspired. . . ."

The New York *Post*, in its typical irresponsible fashion, rewrites the obituary from the *Times*. It begins by saying, quite in error, that, "Funeral services are being arranged. . . ." Nobody at the *Post* has bothered to make a single telephone call or check a single fact.

Although I asked Carole to discourage people and not to give out our address, cables begin to arrive in Port Maria.

It is arriving home that I dread. . . .

Thursday, August 28. Sandy, Rory, and I take the flight that had been scheduled for her. It is uneventful except that throughout the flight the three of us are quite conscious of the notion that her stretcher would have been next to us and the nurse would have occupied the other vacant seat.

Entering the apartment, we busied ourselves with unpacking. But then I began to be overcome, for this was the home she had created and her things were all about us. . . .

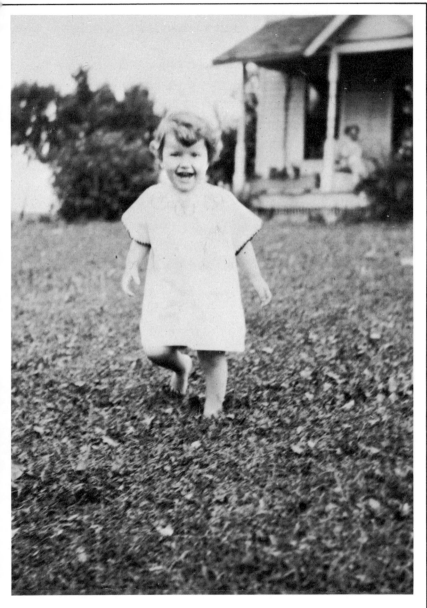

Two years old

And I remembered the tapes and I quickly put one on. And suddenly we were together again, for her rich natural laughter sounded throughout and it was as if she was in the room with us again.

There was the private tape. The one on which she answered my queries for advice. How to handle Rory's education? What do we do about the children and money? And so on, and so on. Every answer so sound, so logical, so precise. And there was a commentary for her unborn grandchildren on the evils of religion. And one on the meaning of politics.

The tapes, more than anything, saved me. Within minutes after I turned the first one on, my despair vanished.

I lay awake all night listening to them.

The wires and letters and sympathy cards pour in. I turn away all phone calls and visitors. The three of us want to be by ourselves.

Some of the notes come from the most unlikely people. Leo Schlemowitz, who had done some carpentry work for her: "Mrs. Stuart was a kind and gracious lady for whom I had great respect and admiration. . . ."

A girl, Miriam Seligman, who worked for us at *The Independent* in long ago 1954. "Perhaps you don't remember me . . . I was going to college in the morning and working with you and Mary

Louise—typing and filing, and you were even trying to make me into a journalist. . . . I know it
must be difficult for you to believe this, but despite the intervening years, I've continued to regard
the period with you and Mary Louise as one of
my outstanding experiences. . . . She was so great
that even a brief contact with her provided me
with an indelible memory. . . ."

Cable from British publisher Ernest Hecht, with
whom we always had so much fun. "She was one
of the most wonderful people I knew. . . ."

A sentiment echoed again and again in the more
than one hundred cables, letters, and cards already
received. Many are from people we haven't seen in
a dozen to twenty years. People in all walks of life
whose lives she had enriched with the magic of
her warm genuineness.

From Ted O. Thackrey: "I shall never forget how Mary Louise joined with you to bring new
optimism and an upbeat outlook to me at the
darkest period of my life. . . ."

From Muriel Moskowitz, an *Independent* reader
who wrote: "I felt I knew Mary Louise Stuart
through the love you showed every time you wrote
about her."

From another subscriber to *The Independent*,
John Kinczel, M.D.: "It'll take more than the usual courage at this time and you have more than
the rest of us."

From John Putnam of *Mad:* "You are my friend. Let this simple statement tell all that is needed to be said at this time. Your friend. . . ."

Of all of them, the two that seemed most to reach me were quite contrasting. Wally Porterfield wrote a beautiful three-page letter which said in part: ". . . I handed [my wife] the letter, and she said, 'Oh, poor Lyle—they were so close. . . .'

"You wrote everything there was to say about death, and did it beautifully and truly, one of the best pieces of writing ever, and I wrote and told you so. It was what you wrote in *The Independent* after Mary Louise's operation, and I said you spoke for me too, and I wish I had written it, and after you read it, there wasn't anything more to say about it.

"It's difficult, though, to realize that that lovely, vibrant woman who was your wife is gone. I can see her very plainly that snowy day I was in New York . . . so charming and gracious—and that last is a wonderful word when used properly. . . ."

And a simple note from Jeanne Taber: "Nobody has to tell you what a good girl you had. Just wanted you to know how sorry I am."

I began this piece in "her room" in Bolt House a few hours after her death. I continued it from our apartment in Brooklyn. And all the while I typed I knew that it was too long and probably could use editing. But she was not here to edit. . . .

"People make too much of death," she had said. And she would have been opposed to devoting an entire issue of the paper to her. But this was one issue I had to write . . . for the children and for myself. It is the only issue ever devoted to a single subject and she was the most important subject in my life. . . .

There are the tapes, which make it seem that she is with us again. There are the movie films and the photographs and the precious letters. And there are the thousands of memories—a quarter-century-full of them.

The beautiful smell of her and the gentle sound of her are fresh about me. And I can close my eyes and see her adorable face and it is twenty-four years ago and she is walking toward me on High Street in Columbus, Ohio, her arms pressing her schoolbooks against her breast . . . walking toward me, my beautiful redhead, smiling her warm beautiful smile at me.

AFTERWORD

More than two years have passed since she died.

Many of the friends and acquaintances who sent me condolence notes about her have died.

I, like T. S. Eliot's Webster, am "much possessed by death" and "see the skull beneath the skin."

We all die. We all return to the earth from which we sprang. And, as those who knew us die too, no trace of us remains, even in memory.

The concept that we did not exist for billions of years is acceptable to us. But the concept that on death we shall cease to exist forever is so frightening to most humans that thousands of religious witch doctors of one kind or another have collected billions of dollars with the promise that there is life after death.

Mary Louise was too thoughtful, too knowledgeable, too courageous to cling to such deceptive nonsense.

The old world, the world she and I knew in our love, is rapidly passing into history. Large cities with safe streets, clean air, and clear waterways are no more. Colman McCarthy describes humans as "a ripple in the contour of evolution . . . doing what no other species has ever done—quarreling with Nature. It appears that man's presence on earth will be nothing more than a brief guest appearance."

Some months after her death, I flew to Columbus, Ohio. It had been twenty-five years since I'd been there.

Things have changed. The Deshler-Walleck Hotel in the very heart of the city had been torn down to be replaced by a parking lot.

The university rooming house where I had shared an attic with two students while I worked as a newspaperman was no more. The house where Mary Louise had roomed at 63 - 18th Avenue had been replaced by a large, modern brick structure.

High Street was something to see. The Ohio State University student body had rioted and smashed almost all the store windows for blocks and blocks. Many were still boarded up.

I wandered to Mirror Lake. Then to the large green where a student rally was taking place. When they made a pitch for funds I made a substantial contribution of money because I knew she would have wanted me to.

There are still a few—very few—familiar landmarks. Larry's Bar is still there—where I had first socialized with the Olsons who introduced me to Mary Louise. So too is the Parker Photo Studio, where she had posed so I could have a current photo of her while she was in Columbus and I was in New York.

The Jai Lai restaurant, where we'd had our first meeting, is still considered one of the best in the city.

I rented a car and drove to the farm outside of Milford Center. The scene could have been a pastoral painting. Everything was still and clean and green and beautiful.

I could imagine her as a child on its lawn or picking thistles ("Dad paid me a penny a hundred.") or driving a tractor or waiting for the school bus.

The next fall, Rory and I and her sister Eileen flew to Dayton. There we were met by her Uncle "Doc" (David Mason), who drove us to the farm. ("I used to tell the children in school he was my millionaire uncle—and I believed it. It was during the depression and every Sunday he visited us and he'd bring a big bag of candy and always give me a nickel or a dime.")

After spending a while at the farm, we drove to her grammar school and then to Byhalia, where the family had lived before moving to Milford Center. We drove through Marysville, where she'd played in high school basketball tournaments. And we visited the high school. Rory collected black walnuts that had fallen from the trees.

I visited Sandy in Los Angeles. On the drive from the airport we talked about Mary Louise.

"You know, Daddy, I liked her better than I liked you. When I was at the University, I used to rave about Mom to all the girls in my dorm. They just couldn't believe anyone could have a mother who said and did the things she did."

Sandy and Rory are unusual people. They have an inner confidence and serenity that obviously came from her.

On one occasion, a group of us were talking about the irony of someone with so much to live for, dying so young.

"I wonder what she really wanted out of life," I said.

"I know, Dad," Rory said. "I asked her about a year ago. She said her idea of a good life was to enjoy each day—to have fun. She said she was having lots of fun."

Shortly after she died, some close friends were concerned that I might take my own life. On one of the taped conversations we made when she knew that her death was imminent, she remarked that it would be a "coward's way" to commit suicide—certainly before the children were grown and settled. After a few years, she said, you might very well find that you were enjoying the life you were living.

She could not know that I would have no wish to escape from the past and that my most pleasant moments would be spent in remembering her and dwelling on our time together. . . .

Dr. Albert Ellis visited our home in Jamaica. On the way to Boscobel Airport, he asked me what I planned to do with the balance of my life.

"Nothing special," I said. "Just live."

"Mary Louise was a very rare person," he said. "You meet maybe one or two or maybe three rare people like that in your entire life. But do you know what I'd do if I were you?"

"What?"

"I'd search for another Mary Louise. Even if it meant meeting thirty thousand women. I'd make that a quest."

"I've known a few dozen women since she died. Many have been very attractive and many have been very nice but when they're in the room with me, even when they're standing one foot away talking, I sometimes feel totally alone. I can't lose myself in new relationships. I've tried. You've got to come up with something better than that."

But he had nothing better to come up with.

When Sandy was eight and Rory a few months from being born, I found a cute note in our mailbox one day. She had written: "It has been a long time since I wrote you a love letter. So now I am. I love you."

Every time we spoke on the phone, our conversation would end with, "Goodbye, I love you." And each evening, before we went to sleep, we would both say, "Good night, I love you."

How beautiful it was once: the rich chance that brought together a girl from an Ohio farm and a boy from Brooklyn—so perfectly matched—so much in love they seemed born for each other.

In a letter to me a few months after her death, and before my first Christmas without her, her sister, Eileen, wrote: "I wish there were any magic words I could write you . . . but I don't know any. All I know to do is to thank you for having made Mary Louise's life so rich and full and vivid and happy that her passion to live was undiminished when she died.

"I hope knowing that she loved you so much, and would be loving you now and forever if she only could, is of some solace to you. . . ."

In the long run, nothing matters. Nothing. Not "fame" or "wealth" or "power" or "health." Nothing. Nothing. It is all a grand illusion—a part of the bitter tragic joke as the ephemera we label "life" races past like a leaf on a riptide.

In some species of birds, when one dies, the mate leaves the flock and waits to die.

No other bird can replace the mate.

And so I live out my life, warmed and cheered by the memories of her, feeling sometimes that she is a part of me and I am now both of us.

And I wait.